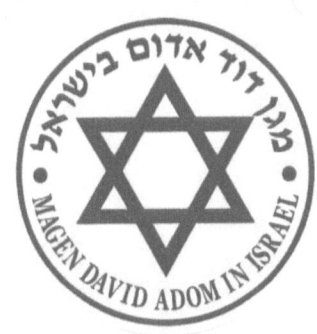

Side by Side with Heroes

Stories of an Ambulance Medic in Israel

Sara R. Ahronheim, MD

Copyright © 2022 by Sara R. Ahronheim, MD

2022 Yellow Wood Books

http://saraahronheim.com

The events and information in this book are true and complete to the best of the author's knowledge. Names and identifying details of individuals in this book have been altered to protect privacy, except in the cases whereby permission was granted to the author.

All rights reserved. No portion of this book may be reproduced in any form without written permission from the publisher or author, except as permitted by Canadian copyright law. No part of this publication may be reproduced, stored in a retrieval system, or transmitted in any form or by any means, electronic, mechanical, photocopying, recording, or otherwise, without the prior written permission of the publisher.

Cover design by Jennifer Stimson

Cover image by Sara R. Ahronheim, MD

Interior formatting and design by Sara R. Ahronheim, MD

Proofread by Sohini Ghose

Issued in print and electronic format

ISBN ISBN 978-1-7386566-0-8 (print)

For Mom, Dad, Divvy and Annie, who watched me run to distant lands and loved me anyways.

For Elie, Cloe and Moe, who prefer to keep me close (the feeling is mutual).

Whomever saves one life, it is as if they saved a world entire.

-The Talmud

Contents

Acknowledgments	XI
1. Code Orange	1
2. History of MDA and the Overseas Volunteer Program	4
3. Introduction	8
4. On the Way	12
5. Settling In	15
6. Welcome to Haifa	19
7. Jerusalem and Back	23
8. Twists and Turns	28
9. Sparkling Summer Days	33
10. Interlude - Home	41
11. Music in the Airport	45
12. Joy in Jerusalem	47
13. First Shabbat	54
14. Moving In	61
15. MDA Jerusalem - Day One	66
16. Filling the Spirit	70
17. Eilat	76
18. Pigua - Kiryat Menachem	81
19. Chanukah and a Birth	85
20. Love In, Love Out	91
21. Dichotomy of Home	97

22.	Waiting for War	102
23.	Gas Masks and Monsters	108
24.	Land of Cats, Doves and Nightmares	114
25.	Best Decision of my Life	121
26.	Snowstorm	127
27.	Interlude - Home	131
28.	A Dream Fulfilled	135
29.	Chamsin	136
30.	May All Your Dreams Come True	142
31.	Pesach in Tekoa, a Lone Soldier, and Murder	145
32.	Choose Your Own Adventure	150
33.	From Sorrow to Joy	152
34.	Smoke and Flames	157
35.	Prayers for Noa	161
36.	Time Stops	165
37.	Sunshine, Chaos, Rainbows, Darkness	174
38.	Death, Birth, Death, Birth	178
39.	Terrorist Transport	185
40.	Epilogue	190
Glossary of Terms		193
Index of Piguim Mentioned		209
About the Author		211

Acknowledgments

I would like to express my sincere gratitude to the heroes with whom I worked side by side throughout my time at Magen David Adom in Israel. Everyone who welcomed me, taught me, worked with me, laughed with me and cried with me — youth volunteers, overseas volunteers, Bnot Sherut, seasoned ambulance medics, paramedics and doctors — you showed me true grit and lit my way. Yael Quinn, Yudah Stein and Aryeh Jaffe: your hospitality, guidance, and teaching allowed me to feel like I could truly tackle the hardships of life in Israel and ambulance work. Dudu Hazanovitz, Boaz Alinson and "Benji": you three are the ones I truly considered my partners at MDA. Your ambulances became safe spaces for me; I will never forget your friendship and mentorship.

Gill Presner, Susie (Sekel) Delman, Judy Zlotnick Birnboim, Chaim Link and all the friends that became like family during my time at MDA and Pardes — thank you, for the adventures, joys and experiences we shared. I will always look back fondly on Shabbat dinners, tiyulim, nights at the cafés and restaurants in Haifa and Jerusalem, and all the moments we had together. Chen Levin — one of my dearest friends, thank you for opening your home to me when I had nowhere to stay, and letting me crash on your couch until I found a place to call home. I'll always remember that kindness.

Todah Rabah to Yonatan Yagodovsky, previous Chief Trainer and Deputy Director of MDA Jerusalem, as well as to Vicki Angel, previous Aliyah Program Coordinator, who provided me with golden nuggets of information about the early days of the Overseas Volunteer Program. Todah as well to Avner Bar Hama, previous Shaliach in Montreal, without whose first steps the program would never have begun. Todah to Yochai Porat, z"l, who solidified my interest in joining the ranks of overseas volunteers at MDA; it was an honour to have met you. Thank you to all the previous MDA overseas volunteers, who answered my calls for information at the outset of the creation of this book.

Thank you to my beta readers: Dr. Heather Gooden, Dr. Jennifer Vassel and Eric Benzacar. Given that I consider myself terrible at self-editing, your honest feedback was invaluable. Thank you to my patient cover designer, Jennifer Stimson, who was always available to make adjustments. I am grateful to Sohini Ghose, who proofread my book and gave it the final touch-ups it needed. Thank you to Michelle Kampmeier, for agreeing out of the goodness of your heart to give my book a quick look and suggest the best type of editing it required. I was lost and you helped to steer me in the right direction.

Todah rabah to all the diverse peoples of Israel, for opening my eyes and heart to customs, traditions, flavours, smells, music, languages and more, that I was blessed to encounter during my time surrounded by all of you.

To my patients: you taught me about human nature, strength, resilience, triumph, fear and sorrow. You formed me like play-dough, into the physician I have grown to be. You trusted me with your stories, as much as you did with your bodies. I can only hope I have described you faithfully.

Finally, thank you endlessly to my family: my parents, sisters, husband, children and dog. Without your constant support and love, this project would never have grown wings to soar.

1

Code Orange

"Trauma Team to the Trauma Room!"

"Trauma Team to the Trauma Room!"

September 13, 2006: My senior resident and I hurled ourselves down the stairs at the Montreal General Hospital and ran together to the Emergency Department. Entering the trauma bay, we were told that a Code Orange was underway — a multi-casualty incident. Just down the road, a shooter had opened fire in the cafeteria at Dawson College, a school I had attended many years before. It was unclear how many victims we were expecting, but it was certain to be an overwhelming number. I was a third-year medical student, on my first rotation of clerkship, and one of the first people in the room.

Standing there, gloves on, waiting for the stretchers to roll in, something happened. Time slowed. My heart rate slowed. My vision cleared. My mind opened itself like a rose, blooming, ready, not afraid. It was time. I had been ready for this since Israel. I looked around me, as the rush began, and dove right in. So many people were yelling orders, dividing tasks, assigning patients. A group of emergency residents were lined up on the wall, waiting to be told where to go, what to do. I just grabbed the nearest patient and started my trauma assessment. I felt sure, I felt directed, I felt I was exactly where I should be.

That day was one of the best and the worst of my medical training. I saw tragedy, I felt my young patients' pain, I heard the desperate cries of family members searching for loved ones. And yet, through all the chaos swirling around me, I felt centred. In those moments, I felt a sum total of all the learning I had gathered — not in medical school, but on ambulances speeding down sun-baked streets, and at smoky ruins of exploded buses where nightmares gave me the tools I now carried into my career as a future physician.

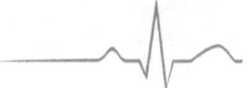

May 8, 2016: While working as an attending Emergency Physician at the Jewish General Hospital in Montreal, I was having a pretty reasonable day. My shift in the acute stretcher zone, having just finished, was busy, but not overwhelming. The purple light went on suddenly, flashing in the bank of lights placed strategically over every room, signalling that a patient was being brought to the resuscitation room (Resus). Glancing up at the board, I saw the name of someone I cared about immensely, a teacher from years ago.

Hurrying over, I saw a physician from an outpatient clinic pushing a stretcher into Resus — something unheard of, as usually it's the job of an orderly to wheel patients around — so clearly this was very urgent. Sitting on the stretcher was my beloved teacher, clutching her head in agony. Another Emergency attending physician greeted them in the room, and began care. The next few hours were devastating, culminating in the brain death of this incredible human being. I spent much of that time comforting her sister in our family room, while inside my heart was breaking. This teacher was there for many of my significant life events. She taught me and guided me, blessed me and supported me. She was there at my Bat Mitzvah at age twelve, she sat beaming at my wedding, and she cradled and blessed my infant daughter at her baby naming.

Losing such a special mentor shattered me, broke my spirit and stole my faith. A faith I had nurtured in sunshine and snow, candlelit desert nooks and hikes to crashing waterfalls. The time I spent living in Israel was the most spiritual time of my life, and yet, in those moments of watching her suffer, it all crumbled before me. I am still sifting my way out of the ashes of my beliefs.

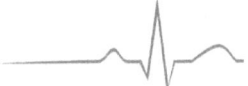

April 11, 2022: I sit, resting in the spring sunshine on our back deck, watching the kids and the dog chasing each other rambunctiously through the muddy backyard. I see my preteen daughter, hair flying, tall, willowy and lovely, as she laughs with my seven-year-old wild child of a son, who asks philosophical questions and loves with all his brave little heart. My strong, capable, handsome husband is grilling dinner on the BBQ and preparing the hot tub for a late-night soak after the kids are asleep.

Idyllic, it seems. Joyful. Peaceful. And it is. But this is an existence I have worked hard for, and one that I know I deserve. This is a moment I used to long for with all of my soul, before I knew it would be, before I was certain.

Israel in 2002, twenty years ago, formed me into the woman, physician and mother that I am today. The people, places and experiences in that time moulded me, trained me, grew me into someone who doesn't give up, someone with grit and the fortitude to do what I have to do every day. The devastation and the passion I experienced back then, I carry forward into my work, my children, and our future.

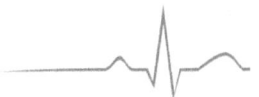

2

History of MDA and the Overseas Volunteer Program

Magen David Adom (MDA), as we know it, is the Israeli national ambulance service. The primary objectives of MDA are defined in the Magen David Adom Law, passed by the Knesset (Israel's Parliament) in 1950. These objectives are to provide pre-hospital emergency medical services, to provide the country's blood services, and to assist the Israel Defense Forces (IDF) during times of war.

Dr. Moses Erlanger, a Jewish ophthalmologist in Lucerne, Switzerland, conceived the idea of MDA in 1915. He created MDA in order to help Jewish wounded soldiers and prisoners of war during World War I (WWI). In 1918, MDA was established in the USA and expanded to Canada, England and Tel Aviv. After WWI ended, MDA was dismantled as the need for a Jewish rescue organization faded.

A dozen years later, on June 7, 1930, MDA was founded — again — in Tel Aviv. It was formed out of necessity, due to the Arab riots against Jewish settlements. The initial first aid course in Israel provided by MDA was held in September 1930, and was taught by Dr. Meshulam Levontin. A total of seventy-three paramedics graduated, and in January 1931, MDA rode out on its very first ambulance call in Israel. By 1933, a branch of MDA was founded in Haifa, and in 1934, the Jerusalem branch opened. The first meeting of MDA associations across Israel was held in the new home of MDA Tel Aviv in 1936.

World War II (WWII) brought misery to Tel Aviv, when the Italian Air Force bombed the city. Thankfully, MDA had trained 50 physicians and 400 nurses and volunteers; they treated 932 civilians after the bombing.

After WWII ended, MDA sent support units to European countries to help treat the Jewish survivors of the Holocaust.

The MDA Law was enacted in 1950 after the establishment of the State of Israel in 1948. This law legally recognized MDA as Israel's primary emergency and rescue organization, which should have allowed MDA to join the Red Cross organization. Unfortunately, this did not happen until 2006 because of disagreement over MDA's Star of David symbol.

Today, MDA operates 169 stations across Israel and uses about 1900 vehicles (ambulances, Mobile ICUs, helicopters, 4X4s, off-road vehicles, Mobile Mass Casualty Incident units, command and control vehicles). Medical teams are made up of individuals with various levels of training.

MDA is unique as an organization because it relies heavily on the use of volunteers to staff its medical crews. High school students, from the age of fifteen, make up the foundation of MDA. Students are trained as first aid responders, and often use their experience at MDA as their high school "Personal Commitment" assignment. Along with the students, there are many *Bnot Sherut*, or National Service volunteers. These are generally young, religious women who work at MDA instead of joining the army for the compulsory two years of service. Every Israeli, at the age of eighteen, must complete twenty-four months (women) or thirty-two months (men) of military service. There are exceptions to this on the basis of religion, background, or for medical reasons. *Sherut Leumi*, or National Service, is an option for religious women who choose not to serve in the army. They essentially complete a two-year professional internship, that could eventually become a career path.

Aside from students and *Bnot Sherut*, the ambulances are staffed by Emergency Medical Technicians (EMTs), Senior EMTs, paramedics and physicians. A specific colour stripe on the sleeve of the uniform denotes each level of certification (red for first responder, grey for EMT, blue for Senior EMT, orange for paramedic). EMTs also serve as ambulance drivers. Generally, the *Lavan* (white) ambulances are staffed by an EMT and one or more first responders, while the *Atan* (advanced life support ambulances) are staffed by an EMT or senior EMT, paramedic and first responder. The *Natan* (Mobile ICU) crew is made up of an EMT or senior EMT, paramedic and physician, as well as a first responder.

In 1991, shortly after the end of the first Gulf War, the leaders at MDA Jerusalem were approached by a *shaliach* in Montreal, Avner Bar Hama, about an idea he had to send volunteers from Canada to Israel to volunteer at MDA. The group at MDA Jerusalem was excited about this opportunity and agreed to help set up this program. The founders of the program were Vicky Angel, Aliyah Program Coordinator, Avraham Halbersberg, MDA Jerusalem Regional Director, Yonatan Yagodovsky, Chief Trainer and Deputy Director of MDA Jerusalem, and Eli Jaffe, MDA Volunteer Coordinator. The Jewish Agency took responsibility for registration, accommodations and the day-to-day needs of the volunteers. The group at MDA Jerusalem sent Mr. Bar Hama the sixty-hour basic EMT curriculum, and verified that the St. John Ambulance curriculum used in Canada met most of the requirements for MDA.

The pilot program was launched in the summer of 1991, and ten McGill University science students participated. They each had basic knowledge of Hebrew, passed the training in Montreal, and flew to Israel to complete a final round of training given by Mr. Yagodovsky. The students were housed at the new immigrant absorption centre in Jerusalem, and spent two months volunteering at the Jerusalem station. Since the initial pilot was immensely successful, the program continued in a similar fashion for the next two to three years.

As demand increased, the program began to gain traction, and it was opened to participants from other countries. These participants received training once they arrived in Israel by doing a ten-day course at MDA. They, in turn, volunteered for six to seven weeks. Soon, the program began to receive thirty to fifty participants each summer, and it spread to other cities such as Tel Aviv and Ramat Gan. The volunteers had such great experiences that they went home and motivated their peers to join the program, and it continued to grow.

In the late 1990s, Yochai Porat took over as Program Coordinator. Yochai was well-loved by the volunteers, as he became a friend and confidant, offering personal guidance and information about living in Israel.

Under his management, the program expanded to eight to nine sessions per year, with participants from all over the world. Within seven to eight years of the program's inception, from hosting ten students, the program had grown to over 200 participants yearly. By 2019, prior to the Covid pandemic, the program was hosting 500 to 600 yearly participants. During the pandemic, the numbers shrank, but the program continued with 150 to 250 annual participants.

Sorrowfully, on March 3, 2002, Yochai was murdered by a Palestinian sniper during his reserve army duty. Yochai had run out to provide assistance to injured soldiers and civilians, and instead he himself was gunned down. That summer, the program that he so loved and nurtured was named in his memory, and is now called the Yochai Porat Overseas Volunteer Program. The program continues to thrive and attract volunteers from across the globe.

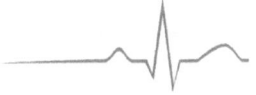

Introduction

February 19, 2022

I am finally here, and I'm so glad that you are as well. It's taken me twenty years to find this moment, and the courage to send these words out to you, the reader.

Today, I am a successful, though exhausted, Emergency Physician at the tail end of the COVID-19 pandemic. I live in Canada, balancing often difficult shifts with the life of a busy mother to two young kids. My vibrant children and adorable puppy fill my life with joy (and my ears with noise), while my triathlete husband has settled into the role of stay-at-home dad. My parents live close by, in the house I grew up in, and my sisters and I remain close.

Back when I wrote the book you are holding in your hands, I was a twenty-three-year-old idealist. I had just finished an undergraduate degree in wildlife biology at Queen's University, where I spent summers researching songbirds in the forests of Pennsylvania and studying Shakespeare and anthropology for fun. I was ready for an adventure, and desperately wanted to experience more out of life before settling into a life in medicine.

I had wanted to be a doctor from childhood, growing up with paediatricians who always talked about medicine at the breakfast, lunch and dinner table. I was that kid who insinuated herself into any first aid situation, from a sprained ankle on the baseball field at summer camp, to an old lady having chest pain on the subway. In university, I served on Queen's First Aid team, and dipped my toes in a world of healing, mixed with thrills and adrenaline. Emergency Medicine was my dream, and first response was my gateway drug.

I first learned about Magen David Adom, the Israeli national ambulance service, when I was a kid at sleepaway camp in 1992. We sat cross-legged on the sweet-smelling grass in the warm sunshine and listened, enthralled, to the stories some counsellors shared. They were among the first batch of Canadian students who had flown to Israel to give their time as first responders at MDA. The memories they shared with us that summer lit a fire in me, and created vivid hopes and dreams that I carried with me until my turn came, ten years later.

In 2001, I took part in an event at a Kosher restaurant in Montreal, where an engaging, warm young man named Yochai Porat was speaking about the MDA Overseas Volunteer Program. He described to us how university-aged young people from across the world would go to Israel for two months to work as volunteer medics. On arrival, the group would take a one-week crash course, including learning the Hebrew vocabulary for ambulance work, and then disperse in small groups to villages and cities across Israel to pick up shifts on the ambulances. Interest in medicine mixed with a love of Israel, and inspired hundreds of us to hop on the next flight.

Yochai was the life force behind the program, and an inspiration. Tragically, not long after we shook hands at our meeting, Yochai was killed by a sniper while in the Israeli army reserves. He was shot while he was trying to provide first aid to fallen comrades and civilians who were under attack; his selflessness and altruism exemplified the very program he had represented. In June of 2002, the year he died, I boarded a plane and flew toward a destiny I had wished for over so many years. Little did I know just how much it would change me.

My first summer in Israel, I lived in Haifa at a new immigrant absorption centre, in a small, hot, smelly apartment with two women from my course. We spent our days working ambulance shifts, roaming around the city, lying on the beach and having the time of our lives. Upon completion of the summer, I didn't want to leave. Instead, I flew home for a couple of months, packed up my life, and moved back to Israel for another year. I spent that year wrapped up in the most amazing experience of my life, living in Jerusalem, volunteering again as an ambulance medic while also at a school part-time learning Jewish studies.

Israel in 2002 to 2003 was in the throes of the second intifada. This was an uncertain and often frightening time to live in Israel, with terrorist attacks such as shootings and suicide bombings being common occurrences. It was also the opportune time for me to go there, as I felt strongly connected to the land of Israel and its people. I felt caught up in a wave of destiny, as if it was my duty to give my knowledge, heart and courage to my country that was suffering. I wanted to immerse myself in the study of medicine and in the land of my ancestors. On my way there, I stopped for a week in Switzerland. I had travelled there before and craved the peace and beauty of the country. In the fresh mountain air, I found separation between my life as a hard-partying and hardworking student in a peaceful, at times boring country, and a soon-to-be-hatched fledgling first responder in a country essentially at war.

These stories that I give to you are raw. I wrote them as diary entries and email journals that I then sent out to friends and family. Some are emotional, and some may feel very disconnected. Being an ambulance medic in a tumultuous time, as a young person with no actual experience of death and suffering, my words, at times, might feel callous. I saw a dead person for the first time, held my hand to a gunshot victim's bloody chest, and didn't write about how I felt. I just described the scene, the excitement of it, the rush. I didn't delve into my soul, and how these moments changed me. Why? Because in those moments, I couldn't let down the walls I had carefully constructed around myself. I didn't know yet how to handle the reality of life and death; the fear, the carnage, the truths of it all. As an Emergency Physician who balances these things daily now, I have found a way to integrate and process the pain of those I treat. Back then, I was so young, and not ready. You will see, as the stories go on, the development of the eventual physician's mind. You will see the range of feeling I finally found working as a medic in a time of blood and fear, in a country of warmth, beauty, and wilderness.

Please see Glossary of Terms for clear interpretations of Hebrew and medical terminology, as well as descriptions of Jewish traditions and holidays mentioned throughout the book.

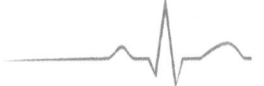

4

On the Way

June 3, 2002 : Switzerland

Hi all,

Not much time.

At the end of May, I left my home in Montreal and embarked on the adventure of a lifetime. At least that's what I hope it will be! I graduated undergrad last year after studying Biology at Queen's University; I spent four years learning about the environment with a focus on wildlife. I wrote my thesis on the mating song of a cute little bird called the Acadian Flycatcher, after studying birds in the forest for months. I also applied to medical school, but didn't get in on the first attempt, so I spent the last year living back at home and taking some extra science courses at McGill. Unsure if I would get into medical school on the next try, I also applied to paramedic school in Ottawa - and I was accepted. However, I rapidly realized that I need some time to make the ultimate career decision. Instead of committing to ambulance work as a job, I decided to fly to Israel and volunteer as an ambulance medic first. If I love it, I'll start in Ottawa in September. If I don't - well - we'll see.

Now I'm in Zermatt, after taking a week in Switzerland before I fly to Israel. I went up on a little train today to the Gornergrat; at 10,300 feet, it is a beautiful place and amazing to see. It was snowing and raining here all day, but then I went for a hike around 6 p.m. just outside of Zermatt, and took a seat on the rock border of the path to watch the clouds magically reveal the majestic Matterhorn ahead of me. I sat there for a good hour, taking pictures and realizing how lucky I really am. Tomorrow I go to the Klein Matterhorn, or Little Matterhorn, at 12,740 feet the highest I've ever been. This is as close to mountain climbing as I'm ever going to get, so I'm taking full advantage of it all. Yes, it's expensive, but who knows when I'll get this opportunity again?

I spent the few days before now on the Swiss Riviera - Lausanne, Montreux, Geneva, and also went up to Gruyères, where they make a delicious cheese of the same name. It was a lot of fun and educational; I hiked up a path fifteen minutes to the village and then walked back down to go see a demonstration of how the cheese is made at the factory. I got free samples and also bought a chunk that I have been snacking on during walks. What a life.

In two days I'm taking the Glacier Express, a beautiful scenic train through the mountains, to St. Moritz, where I'm going to treat myself to the thermal baths and spa. Then off to Zurich, and Israel.

I miss you all; hugs and kisses to my family and especially my little sisters who aren't little anymore - wish you two were here with me.

Love always

Sara

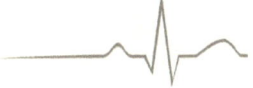

June 4, 2002

Hi all,

I have some time since my feet need a break, so decided to write since I don't know when my next chance will be (maybe in Israel).

I had a fantastic day today; the weather cleared up, and it was bright and sunny at 7:30 when I woke up. I hiked up to the start of a cable car and went up three different cable cars to the top of the Klein Matterhorn. At 12,740 feet or 3883 metres, it's probably the highest I've ever been.

Again, like yesterday, the air was pretty thin and really cold. I climbed up three flights of snowy stairs to the viewing platform, having to stop every flight to catch my breath. At one point, I thought I was going to keel over for lack of oxygen, but I made it.

This place is amazingly devout - there are plaques with portions of the Book of Psalms at the top of the mountain, and on my later hike down I ran into numerous shrines, plaques and crucifixes. I guess it's because people live so close to nature here, and can feel its strength. I stayed halfway up at a stop for four hours, tanning, reading, relaxing, then I hiked down in two hours and the views were absolutely gorgeous.

Being here has settled me, helped me find some peace as I prepare to dive headfirst into a war zone. I am glad I climbed high enough to clear my head, breathe deep and centre myself for the journey ahead.

Time's almost out, gotta run.

Next stop: Israel!

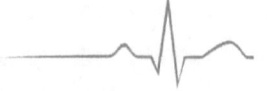

5
Settling In

June 9, 2002 - Chen's place, Jerusalem

Shalom all,

I have arrived!

Here I am, in Israel. Land of milk and honey, as the Torah calls it, symbolizing fertility and abundance. What a trip it's been to get here; on Wednesday I was in snow in St. Moritz, Thursday I was in thunderstorms in Baden, and Friday I walked into a sauna at 40 degrees in Tel Aviv.

I begin this journey in Jerusalem, crashing on a good and patient friend's couch for two weeks until I can find a room to rent. Chen and I have been friends since high school; an Israeli whose family came to Canada, she and I bonded over basketball, downhill skiing and music. Tall (to me, a five-foot-tall woman), with shoulder length, straight milk-chocolate-coloured hair, she is a strong, sensible person with a heart of gold. Chen moved back to Israel and now lives in an apartment in Jerusalem with her boyfriend Ido and their dog. Being an awesome person and friend, Chen offered to let me sleep on her living room couch until I move to my accommodations at the ambulance course.

I've spent my first days wandering the city, in awe of the beauty and history all around. Chen and I hiked to a spring called Ein Sataf, down a rock path and rock stairs which led us to the source, within a dark cave accessible either through an old stone ruin or by crawling through a little tunnel. It was nice and cool in there, and we dangled our feet in the shallow pool. Later we had lunch under the shade of a *Tut* tree, full of fruits called *tutim* that look like blackberries but are much sweeter. We picked them for dessert and climbed back up the hill.

Tomorrow I start my course for MDA, the ambulance service here. I'm so excited, but at the same time nervous. I know it will be exhilarating, but also scary and hard to deal with. I don't know how much I'll get to write, but I'll try. Wish me luck - this might just be the hardest thing I've ever tried to do. But, I am also the happiest I've been in a very long time.

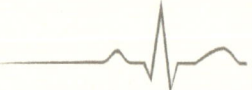

June 10, 2002 - Kiryat Moriah Education Center, Jerusalem

Here I am in the 'burbs of Jerusalem, and I began my ambulance training course today. It's very elementary - some people have no first aid training at all. I'm learning the Hebrew vocabulary for ambulance work, which will be very helpful. Israel has a slightly different way of doing some things, so I have to incorporate those differences into my practice of first response.

The course we are doing is being taught by some superb instructors. First, there's Yael, who is about my age; she is the course coordinator and instructor. She has long, blonde, wavy hair that she keeps up most of the time, speaks perfect English (she was born in the US and moved to Israel with her family at age five) and seems like someone I would like to be friends with. Yudah and Aryeh are two other instructors; both more religious than I am, and younger, but approachable and kind. Neither one of them speaks English all that well (Aryeh hardly at all!) but it gives me a chance to really use my Hebrew.

Overall, it's great here - the people are awesome. There are about thirty-five of us from Canada, the USA, England, Sweden, and Australia. I'm amongst the oldest in the group. There's even a guy here from Montreal, and some girls from Toronto and Ottawa. When the course is over, we will be sent to various cities and villages across Israel, to spend the next two months using what we have learned to help patients on the ambulances. There are eight of us going to Haifa, and we're already planning parties on the beach and renting cars together on free weekends. It's shaping up to be a fantastic time.

Of course, the situation here is as it is. Neil Lazarus (an expert on Middle East politics) gave a seminar this evening on current events in Israel. It wasn't anything I didn't know, but when you're actually sitting in Jerusalem and about to put yourself on the front lines of response in this country, the news hits much harder. Yes, it's a scary time to be here, but I reiterate: it's also the most satisfying time. As most of you know, I've dreamt about doing this for as long as I can remember - I first heard about this program in summer camp when I was thirteen. It's hard to believe I'm finally here. I'm even seriously considering staying here next year, instead of attending paramedic school in Ottawa. It turns out that you can do paramedic training here in Jerusalem, at Hebrew University. I just don't know how I could leave here - last time I came here I said that the next time, I wouldn't leave...but that's not 100 per cent, not even 50 per cent at this point. Just an idea...

I am going to need support, I think, throughout the summer. I hope you are okay with my using this email forum as a sort of cleansing process, to get over my pain. Even though I'm going to have an excellent support network here, I know I'll need that. Writing helps me focus and relax, where talking doesn't always fix things for me.

I have to say one great thing: it's at least a bit cooler here now, maybe 34 degrees rather than 40. It's been years since I was in heat such as this, that makes you sweat behind the ears and in every skinfold possible.

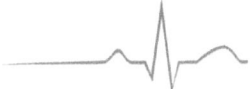

June 18, 2002

Just a quick note to let you know that there was a huge bus bombing in Jerusalem today, only about five minutes from where I am now. We heard the boom. Don't worry, I'm fine, physically. Emotionally is another matter - it's hard enough when we're across the ocean and watching it on TV. To be here, about to write my Magen David Adom exam, with my group and I all wearing our MDA uniforms, and have our instructor walk in and say they had to delay the exam because the bus blew up five minutes down the road - now that's a different story. To know that all the people I've been learning from and working with this past week during the course, who work for MDA now, are all there treating people while I write this email - that's hard. To know that the police and army knew that a bombing was on its way, and had set up roadblocks yesterday to stop it, and still couldn't stop it - that's really hard. Then to walk around this compound in my MDA shirt and have people stop and ask if I'm here to treat the wounded - that's crazy.

So it's harder than I thought it would be, and I don't know how I'll deal with the aftermath of a *pigua* when I actually have to be on the front lines.

I'm okay. Please pray for peace here.

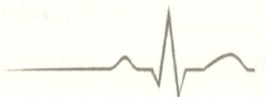

6
Welcome to Haifa

June 18, 2002, 11:40 p.m. - Haifa

Today we had an orientation with our coordinator at the station, got to go in the ambulances and ICU vehicle, learn to use the bed and chair, turn on the lights and sirens.

But I have to say today has been harder than I ever thought possible.

Woke up to a *pigua* with nineteen dead literally around the corner from me.

Had a stressful exam and got certified as an MDA volunteer.

Drove four-and-a-half hours to Haifa. Got to the absorption centre and found a tiny room for three infested with bugs and roaches. An absorption centre is a housing area for new immigrants; it's a really neat experience, as there are people here from all over the world (on my first day I met Ethiopians, Russians, Americans and more). I hope the rooms in the rest of the place are more hygienic than the one they stuck us in today, especially for people here with their families and children. After dropping our stuff, we then went out and had some food (gobbled it up and left) on a small street nearby.

Haifa is on high alert and expecting a suicide bombing at any time now.

Must sleep - shift at 7 a.m.

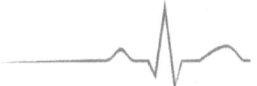

June 20, 2002

Yesterday was my first day on the ambulance; in the whole eight hours I only had one call. We got to the station at 6:45 and our call was a few hours later; a little old lady, who just kept repeating, "I want to make pee-pee!". So we took her to Rambam Hospital. I got to be the primary caregiver, taking her blood pressure, pulse, talking to her, holding her hand. After that, I sat in the station, bored out of my mind.

I got back to the absorption centre at 7 p.m. and just started crying out of frustration. I hope the rest of the summer won't be like this - I felt so useless today.

At least we moved to another room last night, a much nicer place. I am living with two other girls, Becca and Gillian; they are both kind and so far we get along great. Gillian is from Ottawa, so not far from home. Becca has flaming red, curly hair cascading down her back, and Gill has a short brown bob framing her intelligent eyes. We will live together in this small, broiling hot room for the next two months, and share stories of our time on the ambulances.

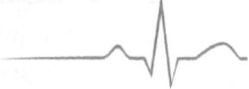

June 21, 2002

My second day on an ambulance! What an incredibly exciting and exhilarating day, with six calls. Most of them were major, and we went with lights and sirens: that was incredible. What a rush! We ended up treating a patient with a spinal injury, another with a heart attack, an old man with high blood pressure, who fainted and hit his head, and a couple more. It was really interesting.

It's so hard living here, though. Last night there was another attack, in a settlement called Itamar in the West Bank. Two Palestinian gunmen infiltrated the village and broke into a house, where they shot a mother and her children in their beds. They killed the mother and three children, and with a security officer. Eight more were wounded. I heard about this last night while I was in a medical clinic; a friend who works near Jerusalem called to tell me. Working for the ambulances, we hear the news before anyone else does, and first-hand. It's terrifying to realize that any day now I could be the one treating terror victims.

Last night we wanted to go out for dinner, and I tried to tell everyone it was a bad idea what with the high alert status that Haifa is on right now. But we ended up having a discussion, and I realized that since I came here to show my support for Israel, I must also support her economically. Going out here also gives moral support to Israel, and we have to live our lives or the terrorists win. They win more by breaking our spirit than by breaking our bodies - and they will never be able to do that if we continue to live for the moment. So we went out.

Have a beautiful and peaceful Shabbat or weekend or whatever you're doing now.

Pray for peace.

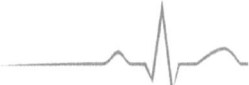

June 26, 2002

Tomorrow afternoon, a few of us are going to Jerusalem to meet up with others from our group, and we're going to spend Shabbat (Friday and Saturday) in the Old City. I'm very excited; as most of you know, Jerusalem is my favourite place in the world.

Here's some fantastic news: I got my MCAT scores today and I made the minimum cutoff mark for medical school! So I'm proud of myself, and hopefully will get into a good school based on these marks.

Things on the ambulance have their ups and downs, as with everything here in Israel. Today was really cool because first I went with three other girls in an ambulance, to a car accident. Our driver pulled up (after driving at high speed with lights and sirens) and all of us drew a collective, shocked, breath. We saw a compact car (or should I say compacted!) and an eighteen-wheeler truck that had rammed into the driver's side of the car and crushed it. The driver was really lucky; no external bleeding or obvious deformities, but lots of pain in the chest and the side where the truck hit his car. We placed him on a backboard and took him to the hospital. Luckily, the patient seemed to be okay.

After we returned to the station, they asked me to switch ambulances to ride with a driver who had no one with him yet. They needed a fluent Hebrew speaker, who could fill out the forms and insurance papers, and they feel that I have really great Hebrew. Usually there is a *Bat Sherut* on the ambulance, so they fill the forms and do primary care. This time I got to do that job - which is so cool! It feels superb to know that Israelis think my Hebrew is *meuleh* - excellent.

On our next call today, we helped a lady with high blood pressure, who was crying hysterically, and her friend came along with us as well. They asked Gillian and me where we were from, and when they found out we were volunteers from Canada, they were so happy. They congratulated us for coming, and thanked us, and said that they were happy that there are still Zionists in the world. When I had explained my reasons for coming to Israel to most of you, I said that one of the most important was to give real moral support to the Israelis by physically being here.

And today I felt that I really am needed.

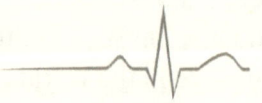

7

Jerusalem and Back

<u>July 1, 2002</u>

I spent the weekend in Jerusalem - it was fantastic. We stayed for free all three nights - two of them we crashed at a friend's house, and one of them we spent in the Old City at a free hostel. Meals on Friday and Saturday were also free. We spent a lot of time walking around places like Ben Yehuda Street, Machane Yehudah Market and the Old City.

I am going to be honest here — many of you want to know what it actually feels like to be here in Israel right now. I'm going to tell you. Sure, it's scary, but bear with me, okay? This is the reality of the situation.

Before I arrived in Israel, some of the worst suicide bombings in the history of the country transpired. In March, thirty people died and one hundred and forty were injured in the Passover Massacre, when Hamas attacked a hotel (via suicide bombing) in Netanya, where Israelis were celebrating the Passover seder. In Haifa, that same month, fifteen people were killed by a suicide bomber in the Matza Restaurant. In May, another fifteen died in a suicide bombing in Rishon LeZion. And just as I arrived in Israel, nineteen people were murdered by a suicide bomber at the Patt Bus Junction, close to our ambulance course.

I have to admit that most of my time in Jerusalem I was nervous - like our last night we went out for pizza at Big Apple Pizza (off Ben Yehuda) and one medic informed us that Jerusalem was on high alert for the possibility of a suicide bombing. I was, needless to say, scared silly. We didn't stay out long. My friends and I had brought our uniform shirts along just in case something should happen, so we could help.

The first night in Jerusalem, we stayed at Yudah's apartment, in the centre of the city (King George St.). Yudah was one of the instructors during our initial MDA course; a tall, thin, freckled redhead, a bit younger than me, with two younger brothers, he speaks fluent French thanks to his parents' Belgian origin. His lovely mother and father welcome ambulance volunteers such as me, taking us in like members of the family, feeding us delicious meals and serving as a support system.

Sleeping on Yudah's couches in the den overlooking the street, a series of six tremendous explosions woke us up at 6:25 a.m. They sounded like gunshots, but much louder, and could only have been one or two blocks away. At the very first one, I was up, off the couch, shoes on and gloves in hand, heading for Yudah's room to grab his medic kit and wake him up. Then his mom came out and told us it's normal, that they blow up suspicious bags all the time — and it was true because we didn't hear any sirens. Moron that I am, I went to the window to look out. The last explosion almost made me fall over in shock. I was shaking all over; I can't begin to describe what went through my mind when I heard those explosions.

On the way back, we took the train from Tel Aviv to Haifa, after taking a *Sherut* to Tel Aviv from Jerusalem. While on the way to the train station, we heard on the news that a suicide bomber had bombed a train in Lod. Lod is only about fifteen kilometres from Tel Aviv.

But listen, these are only the negatives. Being here is like being in a fantastically wonderful dream, even though there are sometimes bad things lurking in the shadows. The wonder and beauty of this place, and the warmth (once you get past the shell) of its people, are gifts beyond belief. I love it here. I hope that one day we can all live here in peace, without having to run around with gloves in pocket and ready to respond to a terror attack.

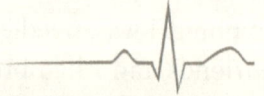

July 2, 2002

Today I spent the day in Banatz, one of our Haifa ambulance outstations. I had the best driver in the station, Motti, as well as a volunteer medic named Ahmad. Working in Haifa is really neat because, especially in this diverse city, Arabs and Jews work hand in hand. Ahmad is an Arab Israeli, and Motti is a Jewish Israeli, and the three of us worked together seamlessly. At Magen David Adom, there is a great mix of individuals of various backgrounds — Jewish Israelis, Arab Israelis, immigrants from various countries, as well as religious and secular people. We all work together for the common goal of treating patients, and the diversity of backgrounds, religious beliefs and ethnicities allow us to relate even better to the people we treat. Today, we responded to nine calls, which is unheard of — usually the max is about five. We went non-stop for eight hours, with a ten-minute break for lunch, and truly enjoyed each other's company.

Partway through the day, as we were driving back to the station, I noticed a man waving frantically at us. I asked Motti to pull over, and we realized the man was pointing across the street at a man lying on the ground, who had been shot literally seconds before, in a robbery. A bystander had his hand on the wound to stop the bleeding, so I pulled on one glove and immediately applied pressure while getting the other glove on with my teeth. I tried to reassure the still-conscious and lucid patient, while Motti and Ahmad took out the chest seal and put it on the wound. I'd never seen a real bullet wound, so I found it very interesting. The wound was actually hardly visible; there was lots of blood all over the chest, but the only way to see the penetration was where the bruising was. There was no exit wound. So there I was, kneeling on the ground, one hand on the chest seal and the other holding the patient's hand, talking to him. I was concentrating so hard on him that I didn't even realize that the mobile ICU truck had arrived, and the doctor and paramedics were helping me. They bagged him with oxygen and started an IV, so then I had one hand on the chest seal and one holding the IV bag until they had to transport. I was so caught up in the patient that I didn't even notice the six police cars with lights and sirens, and the police tape that went up rapidly around the scene, until after I got back to my ambulance.

Phew. Can't believe it. The entire station was talking about the incident all day; it was a pretty neat feeling to know that I was the one with my hand on the bullet wound. He lived, and I hope he'll be fine.

Another call I had today was an old woman who was in lots of pain; her daughter, who was around 70, also came along to the hospital with us. She was crying, so sad that her mother was in so much pain. I did my best to comfort her, and I'm glad to say it made a difference - she thanked me and told me I have a good spirit.

It is very moving to be helping people - it's what I've always wanted to do. And it's even more wonderful to do it here, in Israel.

Have a wonderful, restful, peaceful week.

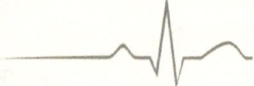

July 5, 2002

Here I am in Jerusalem again, helping to teach the next Magen David Adom course. It's really amazing to be able to help the next group of volunteers - even after only two weeks on the ambulance we have so many stories and so much advice to share. Plus, I love teaching!

Let me tell you about my past few days, and about why I am so tired that I may be unconscious really soon.

Every day when we go to work we are usually running on four-and-a-half to five hours of sleep, and that's fine for my body to function. However, Wednesday we woke up at 6 after four hours of sleep, and did a shift from 7 to 3. Then Gillian and I went straight to the beach, and took in the sun for three more hours. We couldn't swim because it's jellyfish season and the beaches are lined with them. At

6:30 we left and went home to shower, change and pack our bags for Jerusalem. We then left for the mall around 8 to pick up our photos and some gifts we needed to buy. We had dinner there, then went back around 10:30, straight to a night shift. From 11 to 7, we worked the craziest night shift ever! Instead of getting some sleep as we planned, neither one of us slept more than half an hour. I had one call at 11:15 p.m., got back at 1 a.m. and then a driver named Shlomi asked me to accompany him on a transfer call to Tel Aviv. We took a patient to the hospital there (one-hour drive) and arrived back at Haifa station around 3:30 a.m. It was a great drive though; he and I talked a lot and got to know each other. He's only 26 and pretty cool. The first thing he asked me on the drive back was whether I had a boyfriend. Classic. After that I had three more calls, with sleep between 4:15-4:45 a.m. At 7, Gillian and I washed up and caught a train to Tel Aviv, followed by a taxi to Jerusalem. We helped teach all day, and hung out at night with our friends, so we didn't sleep till around 1:30. So how many hours was I awake? 43.5!

Needless to say, I'm tired.

Enough about my life... I'm off to shower and change before *Shabbat*. I'm having dinner with two friends at my cousin Alice Shalvi's house, here in Jerusalem. Alice is a woman I have admired since I first met her; she was close with my paternal grandmother (whom I adored). A true intellectual, Alice is a world-renowned academic, writer, and champion of feminism in Israel and around the globe. I absolutely love being with her and her wonderful family, each time I visit Jerusalem.

Tomorrow we're off to Tel Aviv for the day to have dinner with friends there. Then Sunday we're back here to teach some more, and finally back to work a night shift in Haifa Sunday night.

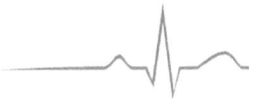

8
Twists and Turns

<u>July 9, 2002</u>

Today I went on a call to transfer a cancer patient from the hospital back to his village, Peqi'in, which is an hour and a half north of Haifa, in the Galil. Peqi'in is a place full of history, first settled in 5000 BCE (!!). It's a diverse place, with a mix of Jews, Muslims, Druze and Christians.

Suleiman, a sixty-nine-year-old Arab great-grandfather, and his fifteen-year-old grandson Fouad came with us in the ambulance. We had a beautiful, scenic ride through mountains and forest to the Galil, and Suleiman and Fouad pointed everything out to me. I rode in the back with them so we could chit-chat.

When we arrived in their village, it was incredible. The village is cut into the side of a mountain, and their house is huge and beautiful. Their whole family was sitting outside waiting for us, and we sat and had juice and freshly brewed Turkish coffee. The Arab-Israeli hospitality is fantastic. They showed me around their house and thanked us so much for bringing Suleiman home. This was my favourite experience on the ambulance by far, because I got to interact with a wonderful group of people and a culture that otherwise I would not have been with. I am so grateful and feel blessed to have had that experience.

Lots more to write, but I have to run.

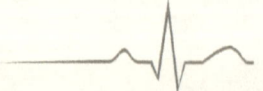

July 13, 2002

Lots to write about tonight. Let's start with the really tough call I had on Thursday, because I need to get this off my chest. I already cried a lot, but writing is always best for me.

First of all, before that: I worked Wednesday night on the Mobile Intensive Care Unit — it was marvellous. We had four cool calls, and the second one was amazing. We responded to a hypoglycemic woman who was having seizures and was completely unresponsive. The paramedic I was with gave her a shot of glucose, and within a minute, she was completely better. It was fantastic to witness him totally saving her life. Unbelievable. She went from almost dead to fully alive, in a minute! I've never seen anything like that in my life.

Now, back to Thursday. I had already been on shift for over twenty hours when we responded to our last call of the day; a car accident, small car vs big bus. The car had rammed, at speed, into the back of the bus. When we arrived, I could see the two heads in the front seats, and I brought the cervical collars out right away. I climbed into the back seat and checked consciousness on both driver and passenger — they were only semi-conscious if that. Both were in a really awful state. I talked to them, but could only immobilize one head with my hands! My ambulance driver, Amir, came and put a collar on the passenger, roughly, so I decided to put the collar on my patient myself so as not to let Amir cause further injury. Amir and the other guy I was working with then proceeded to pretty much yank the guys from the car, giving no heed to the possibility of spinal injuries. It was all I could do to hold my patient's head, and that didn't even help. Amir sent me into the ambulance with the car's driver, my patient, an eighteen-year-old (his brother, the passenger, is fifteen).

I checked my patient's vitals, and he was completely unresponsive. Then Amir brought in the second teenager, semi-conscious, and shut the doors. We took off with sirens blaring, lights flashing, and me alone in the back of the ambulance with two unconscious possible spinal injuries! The fifteen-year-old began to have trouble breathing, and was in lots of pain, and the eighteen-year-old was just completely unresponsive. Finally, as we approached the hospital, he squeezed my hand, then wouldn't let go. When we were getting out of the ambulance, he still didn't let my hand go, and I had to pull away. Once inside, we put them in the beds, and a nurse came and took vitals. But then no one came again. So I was standing between the beds, trying to monitor them, because no doctor showed up the entire half hour we were there. I was holding their hands, talking to them, and Amir came over and told me not to; he made me feel so stupid for wanting to let these guys know that someone cared about them. I turned to the older brother at one point, right before we left, and gave him my hand. He squeezed it, then pulled it to his chest and made signs that he was having trouble breathing. I asked where else it hurt and he pulled my hand to his abdomen. I hope he didn't have internal bleeding.

Finally we left, and I just felt terrible because no one was there with them.

I went back today to check on them, but they'd been sent home already. I hope that means they're okay — I really hope so. The lack of adequate medical care in this case, both on the ambulance and at the hospital, frustrated me enormously.

On a more cheerful note:

Yesterday, five of us rented a car and drove to the Golan, up north. We did a hike called the Yehudiyah, in a deep canyon, by a stream. It took us six hours, and we were carrying so much water and food that my back still hurts. There were amazing waterfalls and pools, and we had to climb down a nine-meter-high ladder into a pool. We also had to climb down handholds in the walls, and go bouldering, to get through the hike. It was spectacular. We climbed up and down cliffs, and up and over many rocks, and swam through many pools. I didn't know I could do something like that. We even brought a raft and floated our bags across the pools. I am so proud of having done it. I've got cuts and bruises everywhere!

On the way back, we stopped in Tiberias for dinner, which was delicious, and this morning we went to Daliyat-Al-Carmel, a Druze village. The Druze are a distinct people who speak Arabic and practice their own religion; they live predominantly in Israel, Lebanon and Syria. In Israel, they participate fully in society and serve in the Israeli army. In the beautiful village located on Mount Carmel, we went bargain-hunting and got some great deals on clothes and gifts. Then we went to the beach and boosted our tans.

Hope you're all well.

July 13, 2002

Thursday my shift consisted of accompanying an ambulance driver named Eran to a *targil* where all the firefighters from Haifa and Hadera were practising at a kibbutz. In 1998, there was a huge wildfire out by Kibbutz Yemin Orde, so they were preparing for a possible recurrence of such a situation. We drove some thrilling back roads and rock paths in our ambulance, which actually stalled once but thankfully recovered. Then we joined the firefighters for a big catered lunch; I was the only woman there the whole morning and thoroughly enjoyed myself.

Let me tell you a bit about living in Haifa. Every day is super hot and humid. That heat can be oppressive, or delightful, depending on the circumstance. For a girl like me whose thighs touch, the heat can mean lots of pain. I wear long ambulance pants most days, and the fabric makes my inner thighs rub raw. I have had to resort to bandaging the skin in that area, in order to protect myself from open, weeping wounds.

However, the beauty of the weather here is that at the end of a working day, or on our days off, we head to one of the numerous beautiful beaches to relax. We jump into the waves, the cool salt water invigorating and cleansing. Often we are there until past sunset, eating watermelon and barbecuing in the sand.

This is the life.

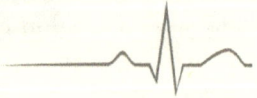

9

Sparkling Summer Days

<u>July 15, 2002</u>

For the past two days, I've been at a seminar here in Haifa. I have a crazy last two weeks planned!

I'm working Tuesday 7 to 3, going to Tzfat for the afternoon, and working 11 to 7 overnight. Wednesday I work 7 to 3, 3 to 11 and then on Thursday morning I leave for Jerusalem. I am doing an advanced medic course in Jerusalem for Thursday, Friday, Sunday and Monday with *Shabbat* in Jerusalem in between. Tuesday we have our MDA volunteer program closing ceremony when we get our certificates, uniform pants and more. Wednesday we leave for a trip to Ein Gedi, near the Dead Sea.

When we get back, that same night at midnight, my friends and I are leaving Jerusalem for a trip to Eilat. We will spend Thursday exploring, after sleeping the entire bus ride. Thursday evening we leave for Sinai, where we will spend time until Saturday afternoon. Sunday, Monday, Tuesday and Wednesday I will do my last shifts, then I leave August 1.

Phew. Crazy, huh? I'm very excited. I'm off to smoke *nargila* with my friends now - for all of you who don't know, that's just flavoured tobacco. You pass the tube around and take in some amazing smelling smoke, and it gets passed around the circle. Meaning you don't actually smoke much, it's just relaxing and a nice way to hang out with friends here in Israel.

Hope all of you are well. I miss you lots.

P.S. Don't worry about me, I'm so happy.

July 17, 2002

I've been working since last night at 11; now I'm on a mobile ICU (*Atan*) shift at Nesher outstation with Gillian and two great paramedics, Assaf and Yaron. The best part about working here is that while waiting for calls, the guys cook! They taught me how to make a delicious Israeli salad with tomatoes, cucumbers, onions, mint and parsley, and they grilled meats for all of us. I will miss working with them, and the fun, social nature of this place.

Last night I worked on a *Natan*, the mobile ICU that also has a doctor on it. I saw my first dead person, a young man who fell from five floors up and was lying in a bloody heap on the sidewalk. It was interesting to see, from a medical perspective, but very sad; such a brief life, and to die alone in the dark morning hours. I wonder if he was conscious for a while first? I hope not; I hope his death was immediate.

Tisha B'Av tonight; twenty-five hour fast. Tomorrow, we leave for Jerusalem to do a medic course.

July 27, 2002

Shalom all,

Lots to write about tonight, not too much time (twenty minutes). I'll try to fit it all in.

Last week I spent in Jerusalem, where I took a course to upgrade myself to Medic status here in Israel, so now I'm officially a *Chovesh*. We learned how to place IVs and practised on each other (ouch!), how to deliver babies (more later) and how to defibrillate someone (you know, shock the heart, like on "ER").

We got our Magen David Adom uniform pants, and hopefully soon we'll get our medic shirts (different from volunteer shirts). We had a special ceremony for the overseas volunteers, where the program was renamed in honour of Yochai Porat. We received certificates — one for the program itself, one for the first responder course, and one for the medic course - as well as T-shirts with the new program name. It was a very touching ceremony: not a dry eye in the house.

Wow, I just realized that so much has happened to me since I wrote last...

I don't think I ever wrote about the best thing that happened to me in my life — and it happened on the saddest day of the year. On Tisha B'Av, the ninth day of the month of Av in the Hebrew calendar, we have a fast day that commemorates the destruction of both the first and second Jewish temples in Jerusalem. It's a twenty-five-hour fast, hard even in North America, let alone in the Haifa heat and humidity. Two years ago I was at the Kotel in Jerusalem, but this year I chose to work on the ambulance instead. I made that decision because I realized that the best way to commemorate a painful time in my people's history would be to help those people through their present pain. So I worked an evening shift at the beginning of the fast.

Barely two hours into it, we got a call (I was working on the ICU truck) to a woman in labour! I couldn't believe it — and I figured she wouldn't give birth till the hospital. She was a beautiful Ethiopian woman, and this was her ninth pregnancy — so it went fast. We got her in the ambulance and within two minutes of driving and putting in an IV, the baby's head appeared. We pulled over, and the paramedic, Yaron, delivered an exquisite baby girl! He let me watch everything from my angle by the mother's head, and I held her hand and helped her through it. He let me touch the baby as she was being born, and I saw the whole incredible process. Amazing! I never thought I'd be so lucky. Then, he cut the umbilical cord and wrapped her up (she was crying by then, sweetie) and placed her on her mother's stomach. He had me monitor her and give her oxygen so she'd start pinking up. The mom was so happy and radiant, and I was glowing. The baby was born to the sounds of "Jerusalem of Gold" and other amazing Jerusalem songs playing on the radio, because of Tisha B'Av. I learned later that babies born on this day are considered lucky, because the Jewish Messiah is supposed to be born on Tisha B'Av. So, the baby felt like a special gift. I was so happy.

Next on my adventure list: the trip to Ein Gedi. My program officially ended on July 25, so the day before, we took a trip to hike in Ein Gedi, by the Dead Sea. It was hot as hell, 42 degrees Celsius, and it felt like an oven. We climbed a steep dry desert mountain in order to get to these amazing swimming holes with waterfalls and ladders to climb down into caves. It was fantastic, and on the way out we ran into an entire herd of male ibex, with huge horns. You can all see my pictures later. Then we went and bathed in the Dead Sea.

A few hours later, my friend Gillian and I got on a bus to Eilat, and spent the wee morning hours (4 to 9) in a sketchy little hostel for about $10. Then we went and sat on the beach, and went out in a boat so Gillian could parasail. It was awesome, and I got really sunburned.

Gotta run soon, but after Eilat, my two friends (Susie and Jen) and I took a cab across the border to Dahab, in Sinai, Egypt. We spent two days there and went snorkelling at Blue Hole. This is an amazing place where the reef is right at the shore and you swim two seconds out over a huge deep hole.

Sinai was great. Really great. Not too scary — only at the checkpoints to get across. We paid about $2.50 to stay each night, and about that much or less to eat each meal. Spent a lot on gifts and travel though, for example, a camel ride to Lagoona, where we swam in pristine turquoise waters. However, some of the men we encountered in Egypt were completely inappropriate and, at times, downright frightening. One offered 500 camels for Susie and me, and one asked me to take a picture with him and then pressed his genitals against me. I felt violated, and we ran out of the shop as quickly as possible. We couldn't walk through the *Shuk* without getting grabbed. Thankfully, there was one shopkeeper who helped us feel safe by sitting down with us and chatting while we perused his *nargila* pipes. He was kind and reassuring.

Gotta run, more later.

I miss you all.

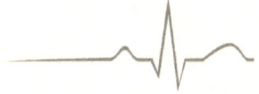

July 31, 2002

Shalom all,

I think this is going to be my last email from Israel. Actually, I know it is. Until October, that is.

I worked my last shifts over sixteen hours in Nesher yesterday evening and overnight. It was great — it always is at that station. The paramedics are really cool, and they are totally laid-back. Unlike at the Haifa station, where people can be less than friendly. In the Haifa station I often felt like a burden rather than an asset as an overseas volunteer, but in Nesher the paramedics just treated me like a regular colleague — with respect. I loved it in Nesher. So I said goodbye to the ambulance this morning, sadly.

We had one interesting call last night — we were called to a penitentiary outside of Haifa, to take a diabetic child molester with heart problems to the hospital. I've never really been inside a jail, and it's pretty scary. It smelled like urine. Yuck. The prison guards were flirting with me, so excited to see a woman, and making some lewd comments. So Assaf (my favourite paramedic) took care of me and made sure I stayed near him at all times. They cuffed the patient/prisoner at the hands and feet when we took him, and a guard came in the ambulance with us. Assaf kept his gun handy as well, and asked me to sit in the front seat while he stayed in the back. It was a pretty wild experience, especially since it was 1 in the morning.

For the past two days, I've been alone here in Haifa. Everyone from the MDA course has already gone back home except me. It's been very lonely, even though I've spent most of my time on shifts. I miss being able to call everyone and talk when I'm bored and lonely!

It was especially difficult this afternoon when I went to the Grand Canyon Mall to escape the disgusting heat. While there, I heard about a big bombing in a cafeteria at the Hebrew University today — seven dead and over eighty-six injured. I spent the next two hours calling everyone I know. It's much harder to deal with a *pigua* here when you're all alone. I was wearing my MDA T-shirt so everyone was looking to me as if I had news. When I got back to the Aba Hushi absorption centre, I went directly to join the crowd in front of the news and got very upset. I had to hold back my emotion because I stick out in my MDA shirt, and all I wanted to do was cry. So I ran upstairs, even in the gross heat, and cried my eyes out. It didn't help much though. I just felt this despairing emptiness inside, like what kind of hope is there and how come I can't help? I felt so helpless sitting here in a sticky room in Haifa, while my friends at MDA were treating bombing patients in Jerusalem.

So that's how I've been feeling today, and it is just been made so much worse knowing I am leaving Israel tomorrow. The only way I can stand to go home is that I know I'll be back here in two and a half months. I know I'm still going to cry like a baby when my plane takes off - I always do when I leave this beautiful place. I don't know if I can ever accurately express what this country is to me, and why I love it so much. It just is that way. I hope at least some of you understand my feelings.

See you all soon.

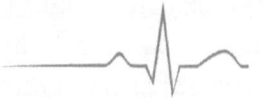

August 1, 2002

Waiting at my gate. Boarding in twenty minutes. It's so hard to think that I'm truly leaving this amazing place. No more Hebrew for two and a half months; hard to believe. Surreal. I don't want to go. When I am not here, I am only half a person. I can't explain it.

Life here is not easy by any means. Not only do you live with a constant level of fear, you also have to build yourself a wall to keep the pain from really hurting you. I learned fast; after the first two days of crying all the time, I built a barrier and tried to become Israeli to some degree. I needed to protect myself from the briskness of Israelis and Israeli society. People here are not easy to deal with; in fact, they're downright difficult. However, once I learned how to get along, I could see through to the warmth within. They might yell at you, push in lines, give you bitchy looks, but you have to understand that the culture is different from what you're used to. I surprised myself and everyone around me by acting Israeli. I feel stronger for it, but I hope that at home in Canada people won't be mad at me for it. I'm going to have to control myself at home, that's all.

Here's the thing: while Israelis are tough cookies, the heart inside is so much more passionate and alive than most elsewhere. I guess a more tender heart needs to be protected with more layers. That's okay, I can deal with it — in fact I'm going to miss it. I love this complexity, and I ache for this way of life. Here you live for each moment, and you fly through the days and nights free. The danger and pain makes living that much more sweet.

Just took off and flew out of Israel. Looking back, I can only just make out the coastline that is receding off into hazy mists. Surreal. Almost doesn't feel as if I was there at all. Sad. I'm going to miss it so much more than words can say.

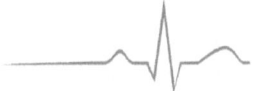

10

Interlude - Home

I left Israel on August 1, 2002 and returned home to Montreal, Canada. This had been the plan since I signed up for the MDA Overseas Volunteer Program, and in September, I was supposed to start paramedic school at Algonquin College in Ottawa. However, after having the most meaningful and wonderful summer volunteering for MDA, I decided that going back to Canada would be merely to prepare myself to move to Israel for a year while applying to medical school. The year in Israel would be spent split between volunteering at MDA in Jerusalem, on an internship program, and studying at a pluralistic Yeshiva, Pardes.

I gave up the acceptance to paramedic school in order to open my heart and follow my dreams.

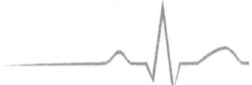

August 1, 2002

Shalom, or should I go back to saying hi?

I'm in between lives here in Switzerland, staying overnight between flights. I had quite a few adventures since leaving Israel... Let's begin with my flight... So I was having a perfectly normal if extremely heartbreaking flight on Swiss Air when I got up to go to the washroom after watching *"Monsters, Inc."*. That's when I heard over the intercom the pilot asking for a doctor or medical personnel. I rushed over (wearing my MDA T-shirt to travel in) and saw a woman lying on the bathroom floor, with a flight attendant kneeling over her. I knelt and began to assess her, and a German doctor working at Hadassah Hospital in Jerusalem arrived to help me. It turned out the lady was three months pregnant with twins or triplets, and was bleeding and having contractions.

We moved her to a lying down position, legs up, near the front of the plane. I took her vitals and assessed blood pressure every ten minutes, and she started to feel better. She only spoke Spanish while the flight attendant spoke German and Italian, the doctor spoke German and Hebrew and I speak Hebrew, French and English. I managed to find a girl to come translate the Spanish into English and German. Phew! I sat next to the lady and comforted her since that's really all we could do. I thought we should have placed an IV and oxygen, but the doc didn't think so. So we just held her hand and kept her calm. She was okay until she noticed my MDA shirt and started to cry while squeezing my hand. She showed me a picture of her niece who was killed while working for MDA. We shared pain.

When it was time to land, I went to my seat, and a short while later, a flight attendant brought me a bag of goodies to say thank you — a big bottle of champagne, a first-class travel kit, and chocolate. They transferred our patient to an ambulance when we landed; I hope she won't lose her babies. When I landed in Switzerland, I found out that today is the National Independence Day. Everywhere they're giving out chocolate and there are tons of fireworks. Each time I hear the booms, I get goosebumps because they sound so much like other bad things and, coming from Israel, I'm quite on edge.

The difference between Israel and Switzerland is so stark — it's like black and white. Here it's so safe, so easy, so nice. People are so polite, so helpful. Life is slower paced. But I love Israel so much more. My flight tomorrow is at 12:55, and I should be back in Montreal at 3 Montreal time. Call me!

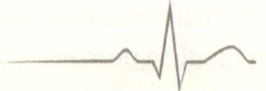

August 2, 2002

Shalom,

I'm home. Can't say I'm too happy about it either. It's just as hot and humid here as it is in Haifa; gross! And my cab driver on the way home from the airport insisted on talking Israeli politics in French for the whole twenty minutes, and ended up coming on to me. So I lied nicely and told him I have a boyfriend in Israel who is currently in the army, which didn't help, as he offered himself for the two months that I'm here, to keep me "satisfied". GROSS!

Finally, I got home and lucky me, my parents had changed the alarm in our house, so the alarm went off and scared the hell out of me. Finally, I worked it out with the company. Once things were settled, I went outside to my backyard to check on my garden - which is beautiful! I picked some cucumbers, zucchini and raspberries, and exchanged insect-human communication with a beautiful red dragonfly that let me get close enough to touch.

It feels surreal to be home. Like it's all a dream, or rather that Israel was all a dream. Only my tan, my braids from Egypt and my pile of luggage remind me that yes, I really did just come home from a summer that I've been craving since I was twelve years old. I really did just live out my dream. And I'm going back for more.

I can't wait to see those of you on this side of the ocean, and I can't wait to see the rest of you in Israel when I get back. I'll miss all of you, especially my incredible lifelong friends from MDA. Keep in close touch, because I need you all more than anything right now to get past the aching inside.

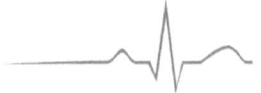

August 4, 2002

Is everyone okay? I hope none of you were near the bus that was attacked on the road from Haifa to Tzfat. Very scary, since a bunch of us took that same bus a few weeks ago. Please write to me to let me know you're all okay, if you're still in Israel. Especially you guys and gals in Haifa: ease my mind and let me know you're okay. Also, those of you in the army — I read that there were a lot of soldiers on the bus. Just let me know you weren't one of them.

God, I wish I had my cell phone and was in Israel to call each of you!!!

Be safe.

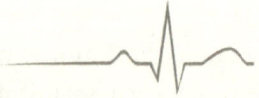

11

Music in the Airport

October 13, 2002

Hey everyone!

It's time once again to begin a new email diary. Tomorrow, (actually, technically today) I leave for a real adventure: ten months in Jerusalem, Israel. At 8 p.m. I fly out of Montreal, and arrive in Tel Aviv around 5 p.m. Israel time. I will volunteer on the ambulances again, a few shifts per week, while also taking interesting courses at the Pardes Institute of Jewish Studies. I'm really excited, albeit a little nervous, as I pack and re-pack and remove things and re-pack them again. Recently, I got a flu vaccine and typhoid vaccine, so I should be well covered, and I'm supposed to be getting the smallpox vaccine when I start working for Magen David Adom.

I have a laptop computer now, so I will hook up to the internet as soon as I get my apartment in Jerusalem. I will be in constant email contact, and also plan to hook up a PC-to-PC phone system where I can call someone else's computer and talk to friends through a microphone-speaker setup. That way I would only pay internet time, not long-distance charges (most of you probably know how I got really badly scammed on my cell phone rental this summer.... never again!). I'll let you know when it's set up, so if you want you can download the same software and we can chat via the computers.

I'll miss all of you, and hope to see you soon when I come back for medical school interviews (I HOPE).

Good night, sleep tight, and in a couple of days I'll be in touch from Jerusalem.

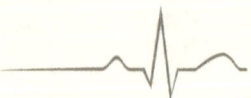

October 13, 2002 - In Toronto airport

Sitting at the gate listening to a group of kids my age singing "Yerushalayim Shel Zahav" with a guitar and flute. You know you're in the right place when the entire group of people sing together; all these strangers being nice and peaceful.

It's great to be flying home to Israel, to Jerusalem. It was raining today in Montreal, but upon getting to the airport, a huge double rainbow spread out overhead. What a good omen. I couldn't believe it, so beautiful; it put my mind at ease.

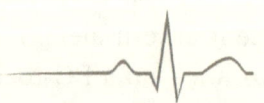

12

Joy in Jerusalem

<u>October 15, 2002 - Gilo, Israel</u>

I've arrived safe and sound in Israel, after flying eleven-and-a-half hours from Toronto. My flight was comfortable because the old lady sitting next to me moved to an empty seat, so I managed to lie down and sleep. My mom's friend Manya and her family picked me up from the airport and brought me to their home. Manya is my mother's oldest friend, her best friend from childhood. They grew up in Montreal together before Manya moved to Israel to marry the love of her life and raise an enormous, constantly growing, religious family. Manya and Benny live in Gilo, on the outskirts of Jerusalem, not far from Bethlehem.

We had a nice dinner and then I sat and read my book (*Black Hawk Down*) until midnight when I fell asleep. I woke up this morning around 6:45 to bright sunshine and little birds hanging out in my window. Realizing I was waking up in Israel gave me mixed feelings, so I went back to sleep until 10:30.

If you want to know the truth, which I'm sure you do, ambivalence characterizes these first twenty-four hours overseas. I've never chosen to be this far away from family for such a long period of time (ten months) and I'm not so sure I'll last the whole time. Last night I actually cried for a while in my room here, and only stopped by telling myself that I can leave whenever I want; I can just pick up and go to the airport, change my ticket and fly home. But that's not what I came here for, to chicken out and leave.

I am here for good reason, and I need to be here. In a few days after I settle in a bit I'll go to Pardes, the school where I'll be taking part-time studies, and set up my schedule. Then a week or so later, after settling into that routine, I'll go to Magen David Adom and set up my ambulance shifts. Hopefully, within a week from today, I'll have found an apartment and moved in.

Back to the real stuff — my feelings: I find myself continually pushing them away by reading, or doing something to take my mind off missing my family. But it's a losing battle; the sadness creeps up on me every few minutes and I have to fight back tears. Probably this is an artifact of my flying for so long and having my body clock all messed up, but I am also just being me. Why do I put myself in these situations, far away from security and comfort and the tranquil home life? I suppose it is because I need that thing called adventure; I need to feel like I'm really alive. But this time around I am here because I feel a duty to be here, and I feel obligated to help my people in a time of crisis. I know coming here is the right thing for me to have done, and I am proud to be here. I need to start my life here, and once I'm in the midst of helping people on the ambulances and learning Jewish studies, I will forget my feelings of being misplaced and alone. My friends here will help me get used to Israel again and the difficult way of being here, and I will put back up that shell I used this summer when I felt so sad at times.

Don't think that I am regretting my decision to come here; I haven't yet been here long enough to make such a judgement. All I know is that I am here, and I will carve a life for myself here no matter how long it takes or how hard it is. I can do this. I am ready for this and this is what I have chosen to do with my skills and training.

I will keep in regular contact but understand that for a week or more I won't have a regular internet account. I may not be able to answer your emails right away, but know that I am thinking of each of you and miss you.

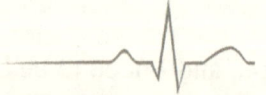

October 16, 2002 - Chen's place, Nachlaot, Israel

Here I am in Jerusalem, Nachlaot, to be exact. After spending my first night in Gilo, Chen picked me up and brought me to her apartment. Now I am sitting on my makeshift bed, glad to be here. It's thundering outside, with spectacular lightning in the Jerusalem sky. Earlier I tried to plug my computer in but was stupid enough to have my fingers on the metal prongs, so I succeeded in electrocuting myself. It was the strangest feeling; I saw the bluish tinge of the spark as I felt the wave of electricity go through my left hand and straight to my heart. I actually felt my heart beat strangely, irregularly, for a couple of seconds, and I was slightly nervous that I'd screwed myself up. But there are no burns on my hand, no entry or exit wounds, and I feel all right now. This happened about an hour ago, so I'm going to stay awake a little longer just to be sure I didn't hurt myself. They say that electrocution injuries can manifest themselves hours or even a day or so later; I hope that doesn't happen. In any case, it was only a second or two of contact before I pulled away. My reflexes are pretty good.

I'm listening to a calm CD I made for a friend on the occasion of her bridal shower. It's relaxing music, or what some of my friends would call "chick music." It's comforting, and reminds me of home and driving in my car. Thankfully, the weather cooled off this evening; the daytime was pretty hot (even though I was sitting in Manya's apartment all day long, it was still humid). I feel a little better about the whole situation right now; being in Jerusalem itself, with a good friend, and getting ready to check out apartments... well, it just makes things easier. I was a wreck last night; really upset, ambivalent, crying. I miss my family, that's for sure, but I can do this. I know I am strong enough to do this.

I got another medical school supplementary application today, which is great. I've gotten one for almost every school I applied to. I'll start working on the application to Rush University tomorrow; it's on paper, so I don't have to use internet time (precious expensive minutes). It's nice to be here now to do the rest of this medical school admissions process. I'm less stressed about it and have my mind on other things, like living! Hopefully, around January or so I'm going to have to fly home for interviews. It would be great if I can schedule them all in a one-month period, but the discrepancy between Canadian and US schools may force me to fly home twice.

So back to the feelings... I talked to Chen for a few minutes today about not knowing if I really want to be here. She said it takes a while to get used to (which I know from this summer's experience) and that she's here for me. I feel so lucky to have Chen to support me - knowing I can talk to her anytime I feel sad or lonely really helps. Still, it's strange to have arrived in Israel after wanting to be here so much, only to recognize in myself a huge element of fear and anxiety. I suppose it is partly the idea of being in a country under imminent threat from Saddam Hussein and all the other Middle Eastern countries, as well as being under constant attack by terrorists within the borders and cities. But truthfully, my feelings aren't borne of this type of fear. Sure, driving down from Gilo today, I felt that being in Jerusalem was totally taking my life into my own hands, but why not? It's my life!

Aside from the fear of dying, which isn't foremost on my mind, I am afraid of loneliness. I am scared to begin my life here, only to realize that this is not where I belong. Sometimes I just look around and can't believe I'm here, because why on earth would I leave a wonderful, secure place like Montreal to come to Jerusalem? Sure, I have many friends and family here, but what about those lonely times when I will sit alone in my room, thinking of my sisters, my mom, my dad? What about when I need hugs and don't have someone to give them to me?

Being twenty-three years old and about to enter medical school (I hope!) I should be able to live here for ten months in relative happiness. In fact, scratch that, I will live here overjoyed, because I have wanted to do this since the first time I set foot on this beautiful land. Yes, I will be lonely, but I can fix that by being with friends and family here. Yes, I will be scared, but fear is surmountable, especially when I will see many people who are more afraid than I, like my patients in the ambulances. When I hold a person's hand and try to stabilize their condition, I will not be afraid anymore because I know I am strong, whole and healthy. I know I am lucky to be here, lucky to be young and free and independent enough to make a life-altering decision to come here. I am happy, and while I miss my family, I know they know I am happy. And that counts for a lot.

Well, I'd better go to sleep. Tomorrow I begin calling around to see apartments. I'll need all my wits and strength for that.

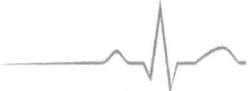

October 16, 2002

Shalom everyone,

I've spent the past day looking into apartments to rent; tonight Chen and I visited two, of which one is promising. The apartment is five rooms, and they're all nice; the room I would rent has its own shower and toilet — a big plus. The downside is that its other occupants are a mother and her university-age daughter; a bit of a strange set-up for me. We'll see — I'm going myself to check out a few places tomorrow while Chen's at school.

Jerusalem is interesting, as usual. I remembered why I love it here. The people are so great for watching; the smells are intoxicating (except the horrific stench of garbage rotting on the corners thanks to a huge strike); and the views are unmatched. Truthfully, though, it continues to be a scary place; there are always helicopters overhead going to places like Beit Lechem (Bethlehem) or Ramallah — I need to get used to that. The buses are out of the question right now due to the threat of suicide bombings, so I'm walking all over town. Chen and I walked down Ben Yehuda Street today to go change my US cash, and we wanted to run down it because it is seriously one frightening place. Having been the scene for some awful terrorist attacks, but also the main shopping street in Jerusalem, it seems overdue for more carnage; I hope it never comes. You really have to watch yourself here, but you just feel more alive for that. I love it here.

Tomorrow I am also going to call Pardes — I left them a message today but we don't have an answering machine here. Pardes is the school where I will take really interesting Jewish Studies courses — I am very excited to go check it out. In a few days, I'll get in touch with the lady in charge of my internship program at Magen David Adom, and try to set up a schedule.

It's hectic here, but a much better feeling than I felt two days ago, when I first arrived! Stepping off the plane, I just wanted to get right back on, but now I am getting adjusted and I feel great. Yes, I still miss all of you, but I am settling in and doing just fine.

By the way, I have a cell phone number so feel free to call (I would be ecstatic to hear from anyone). I can't figure out how to change the voice message or even how to get my messages, so don't leave any! Write soon, but I can't promise to write back quickly.

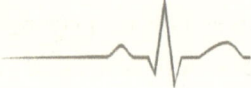

October 17, 2002

I spent the day today wandering around Jerusalem on my own, checking out apartments, visiting a friend and going to see Pardes, the school I will attend starting Sunday. I am amazed that I didn't get lost more than once today. At the end of my day, at sundown, I found myself standing at the end of a beautiful street overlooking a vista with the Knesset (Israeli parliament) ahead of me on the next hill. Surprisingly, Jerusalem is pretty easy to navigate, especially since I speak Hebrew well and can get good directions from people on the street (did I mention yet how NICE Jerusalemites are?). This place is fantastic. I am over my initial ambivalence and now know that this is right for me. I am very, very, very happy to be here and proud of myself for taking this amazing step.

The apartments I looked at today were not exciting. Suitable locations, but each had something significantly wrong with it. One was nice, nice landlady, etc. but the bedroom was unfurnished, it was four floors up with no elevator and there was no den or common room. Another was quite nice, clean, but tiny, especially the bedroom (lots of closet space though!). Another one was just a dump. It's okay though, I have an entire list to call later and some that I'm hopefully seeing tonight with Chen. I'll let you all know when I have an address.

For lunch I met up with Yael, my instructor from MDA this summer; she's really fantastic (Yael when you read this, it's true!). We had a fun time hanging out in her office (very busy lady) and chit-chatting. A funny thing happened: when I was home in Montreal, I was corresponding via email with this guy Adee, who had a cool apartment and was looking for a roommate. We emailed back and forth for a while, but I decided I had to see it before really considering it, so we stopped emailing (I wasn't coming here for another month). Turns out he works in Yael's office. Talk about small countries; Israel is incredible that way. Anyway, turns out he also goes to Pardes. He's really nice, so I got his number and I suppose we'll be in classes together. Too bad he already found a roommate; he would have been a good match for me apartment-wise.

As for Pardes: I went there this afternoon and was really pleased. It's not in the nicest looking area (industrial section of Talpiot), but very accessible and near a great street called Emek Refaim (excellent restaurants, cafes, etc.). The registrar there, Ronit, was really helpful and nice, even recommending a good liberal synagogue for me to attend if I want. I'm starting there on Sunday; we'll see what courses would be best for me at that point. I'm going to be there five times per week (once/day) and work for MDA three to four times per week depending on how I feel.

So it's all working out. I'm so excited to be here!

I miss you all. Write back soon.

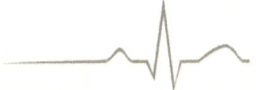

13

First Shabbat

October 22, 2002

Shalom,

I'm all right — nowhere near the horrible bombing yesterday.

Doing fine learning at Pardes, starting MDA again soon.

Can't write much, must go, will write tomorrow. May have found an apartment.

Miss you all.

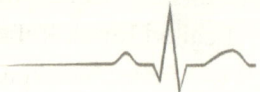

October 23, 2002

Shalom everyone,

I didn't have much time to write yesterday, but I have a few minutes now at this little internet cafe. I had a whole email written out on my laptop, but these computers here won't let me open a floppy disk. Oh well, it wasn't genius in any case.

The bus bombing near Hadera (Karkur Junction) was horrific and I'm glad I didn't have to be on the responding ambulances. I haven't actually started with Magen David Adom yet; hopefully, next week, as soon as the apartment hunt is over.

Speaking of which, I saw a great place yesterday that I will sign for as soon as the roommates give their OK. Two of the people there are students at Pardes with me, and the girl's boyfriend also lives there (he's a rabbinical student). The bedroom is really nice, quite spacious (the size of my room in Kingston during undergrad, I guess) with a window. It has a bed and desk, and the closet space is out in the hall. I'll have to get myself some sort of dresser, maybe an armoire type of thing. We'll see. The rent is reasonable because it includes the city tax already, and they're getting cable internet for the equivalent of about $15 per month per person. Not bad. So hopefully they'll want me as a roommate, and I can move in soon. I've definitely stayed long enough at Chen's house; she's most likely sick of me by now. I know if I was her I would want my space back (so thanks Chennie).

Pardes is great. Turns out I know a couple of the guys there from my time at Queen's University Hillel. The people are really interesting, mostly North American. I'm taking a Talmud/Gemarah class, Modern Jewish Thought, Women and *Mitzvot* and *Tefillah* classes. The teachers are skilled, and I'm learning so much. I forgot how much I enjoyed Jewish learning.

My first Shabbat as a person living in Jerusalem was filled with friendship and happiness, as it should be every week. I stayed with Gillian (from MDA in Haifa last summer) and her parents at the Inbal Hotel (formerly the Laromme — super swanky) because they were here from Ottawa on a United Israel Appeal trip. We spent our *Kabbalat Shabbat* at the *Kotel*, surrounded by hundreds of others. It's a truly special feeling, to be at the *Kotel* and know that I can come to it as often as I wish for ten months! We saw our friend Aryeh (instructor from the initial MDA course); he joined the *Yeshivat HaKotel* boys as they danced down the stairs to the plaza. Each Friday night, the students at this *Yeshiva* dress in white and sing and dance their way down to pray - it's beautiful to see. We watched them for a while and felt the joy inherent in such an evening.

Our friends Yudah and Lior (his brother) came to visit us Friday night after dinner, and that was really nice and relaxing. On Saturday, we walked down Emek Refaim street to Yael's apartment and had a wonderful *Shabbat* lunch with her, her boyfriend Yaniv and roommate Gadi. Thanks Yael! Later, we walked to Aryeh's apartment and hung out for a bit. After saying goodbye to Gillian that evening, I went with Yudah to watch *Austin Powers* at his friend Yotam's house, after first stopping by the clubhouse of Bnei Akiva, a youth group here. The kids there were hilarious, and super excited that I had come from *Chul* purely to volunteer for Magen David Adom.

Before I sign off, I just want to say that I am so happy here. I am proud of myself for coming here, and for getting through this initial phase of confusion and nomad existence. I love being here, and by the time July comes, I'm sure I won't want to leave.

Jerusalem itself is, well, fantastic. I know so many people here, and I love using my Hebrew.

Living here is wild. I love it.

Miss you all.

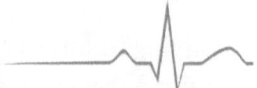

October 24, 2002

Tonight, I had a great time hanging out with Yael. We went to her parents' home in Ramot, outside Jerusalem, and had a delicious dinner. Then Yael dropped me off back at Chen's while she went out with her friends to a play. She's really wonderful; she totally helped me out without any questions. It is so nice to have friends like Yael and Chen, who have been helping me with a place to stay and leave my things.

Vis-à-vis the apartment search — well, that pleasant apartment near Pardes would be ideal, if only the roommates there would make up their minds and call me back! Today I asked them what was going on and they said they hadn't discussed yet but would call me before Shabbat. Yeah, right; it's Thursday night already.

This whole situation is really upsetting me, not only making me angry, but sad. I've been very emotional, almost crying every few minutes these days. I just want to find a permanent place to put my bags, a bed to make with sheets and pillow, a closet to hang my nice clothes and a washing machine to do my laundry. My wish is to move in with people who are friendly and open, who really honestly want to be around me and enjoy my company. I realize that it's a lot to ask for, but I think I am a really cool person who would make a great roommate... why is it so hard? I wish they would just make up their minds so that I could either move in or move on. It's really not nice to leave a person in limbo like this. And I feel like if I call them, I'll seem like a nudge and they'll definitely say no. What to do? Keep shlepping all over the city like a forlorn backpacker or something? My duffle is still with Manya, and I know if I could deal with living in Gilo that I would always have a room to sleep in up there. But it's too far away and the buses out there are just too dangerous to take regularly.

Speaking of which; my bus ride to Talpiot today was scary. As I got on the bus, there was a guard there, watching each person to ensure no terrorists were among us. On the way to Pardes, the bus ride was fairly normal until we got stuck in a traffic jam a block away from my stop. Soon we saw a police car blocking the road, with a police officer checking each car before letting it pass. He boarded our bus, and as he did so, a bunch of us got off. Looking down the street, I saw many police cars and army vehicles, where usually there are only one or two. After classes ended, I came out to have lunch at the mall across the street, and on my way there passed at least four police and army trucks full of soldiers and police officers. There were two security guards at the entrance instead of just one, and guards posted along the side of the mall. I went inside anyway and had a quick lunch before getting the heck out of Talpiot. It was just too unnerving today. There must have been a huge alert for that specific area. Well, I hope they found who they were searching for. Or I hope it was a false alarm.

My day today even started with fear: the sound of what seemed like a dozen helicopters overhead woke me up at 6:00. The noise lasted for a good ten minutes. Living here is definitely not the safest thing; today I truly felt that I am in a country perpetually at war. Nevertheless, I love it here more and more each day.

Even though difficulty is part of life here, and the struggle with my emotions is intense, I consider myself enormously lucky to be living in this place. Jerusalem reminds me each day of the esteem I hold her in, and she fills me with joy by just letting me walk on her streets. The people here surprise me with kindness and passion at least once a day, if not much more, and I learn so much about humanity here.

The shortest moments, the seemingly most insignificant things, kindle hope in me for our united future.

For instance, watching the bus driver and the guard chit-chatting today - two young guys, perhaps my age or younger, playing pivotal roles in keeping our people safe - this is what I mean. The responsibility that weighs on the shoulders of these young men and women is enormous, and I respect them so much for it. Being a bus driver or guard in Israel, and surviving, is truly cheating death every moment; these are the first people to die in a suicide bombing. Every day, these guys must go to work with dread in their hearts, or fear, and most likely pride and determination to protect us at all costs.

Then there are the people on the streets. By the bus stop today there were two homeless people begging, and I just passed them by, ignoring them as I would any beggars in Montreal. But then I was ashamed as I watched a young girl behind me stop and speak to these poor people, and apologize for not having money to give them. I think people here actually respect each other more, even with all the initial *Sabra* hostility and aloofness. Here the people of Israel are bound up in a struggle for existence different from all others we have known in the past. Perhaps we are being strengthened by it in unlooked-for ways. Where else in the world would you find such courage as you do in Israel? I don't believe there is any other place quite like this, my homeland and the forever home of my people. We are here to stay, and no matter how much pain we must endure, we will overcome.

Helicopters, big guns, soldiers, sirens.... these are all part of my daily life in Jerusalem. But lest we dwell on war without recognizing peace where it lies, let me stress this point: while we may have suicide belts tightening about the waist of our country, we continue to push against the noose with love of the Jewish people and faith in our country, Israel. No, we are not anywhere near perfect and there is much healing to be done within our nation, but the goodness I see in my people here will pull us through.

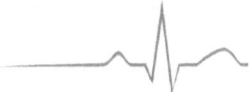

October 25, 2002

Shabbat Shalom!

For those of you who don't know, that is the traditional greeting between Jewish people upon welcoming the Sabbath day. Walking the streets of Jerusalem, and in all business dealings here on Fridays, everyone says *Shabbat Shalom* to each other. It can be loosely translated as "Have a restful Sabbath." This is just another reason I love being here. It's hard to explain why *Shabbat Shalom* is so meaningful to me... but I'm sure many of you feel the same way about this phrase or another.

I have great news to start off my *Shabbat* — I got a call this morning from Chaim, one of my *Chevruta* at Pardes, and one of the people living in that apartment I like so much. Turns out he and his flatmates have agreed that I can move in — so I will do so after Shabbat! Isn't that wonderful? A room to call my own, with a bed I can make with my sheets and pillow. A kitchen I can cook in (albeit dairy, and fully Kosher — which is good), a den I can relax in, a nice bathroom... and intellectually stimulating roommates. Very exciting. I'll send out the address soon so you can all write me letters or (hint hint) send me packages.

In a few minutes I'll be going to Shuk Machane Yehudah to pick up two salads for dinner tonight, yummy clementines (they're green here, interestingly, and we have green oranges too) and flowers. I've been invited for *Shabbat* dinner at my old friend Davide's place in Nachlaot; he and his wife Julia are very sweet and I'm excited. Davide and I went to high school together in Montreal, and ran with the same tight crowd for many years. He is someone who knows me very well, and seeing him here in Jerusalem will be so much fun. Another old friend of mine, Tobi, is coming as well, and I haven't seen her in years. We swam together in swim team, went to school and summer camp together, and have basically known each other forever.

That's the cool thing about Israel, and specifically Jerusalem — this place is a meeting spot for people who have come in and out of one's life. They all end up here somehow, which is fantastic.

Anyway, I should be off soon.

I miss all of you and will write after Shabbat.

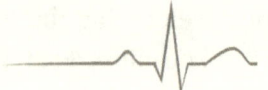

14

Moving In

<u>October 27, 2002 - In my new apartment: 24 Rivka Street, apt.13, Bakaa, Jerusalem, Israel!</u>

Sitting at *my* desk, in *my* room, in *my* apartment (well, not only mine, but still, close enough). I had the most amazing weekend, and this is the best ending to it. Let's begin with Friday night...

My friend Tobi graciously allowed me to stay with her on Friday night for Shabbat. We went to a beautiful *shul* called Mayanot, in Nachlaot, to *daven Ma'ariv* and *Kabbalat Shabbat*. I especially liked it because, although there was a *mechitzah*, the Rabbi came and spoke at the front so that he could see both the men and the women, and we could see him. For the first time in such a *shul*, I felt a part of the congregation, and I felt important instead of invisible. The singing was beautiful and spirited, both men and women lifting our voices up. Davide and Julia were also there; we'd planned ahead of time to all *daven* in one place and then go to their place for dinner. We had the most beautiful, wonderful, warm dinner; the four of us plus two other girlfriends of Julia's. We sang and told stories until midnight.

The next day I went to Shir Chadash, Tobi's shul. I liked it, but not as much as Mayanot. However, at kiddush, Rabbi Shalom Brodt was there, and he invited me for lunch. He was my Torah and *Nevi'im* teacher at Herzliah High School; long time no see. He lives here now and is a well-respected rabbi in Jerusalem. The kiddush was nice; stories, anecdotes of Shlomo Carlebach, and delicious hot kugel. Lunch at the Brodt's was fantastic, with about twenty people there, including Davide and Julia. I didn't leave until 4 p.m. We told stories, ate and sang for a full four hours. I left there feeling very spiritual and ready for a good nap.

I woke up around 5:45 and made *Havdalah*, then went over to Chen's for her housewarming party. That was a totally different experience, a fully *chiloni* evening. It was fun; I met some nice people and had my first experience doing the party small talk all in Hebrew with a guy named Yaakov. Nice guy, attractive, Israeli... the works. I enjoyed trying to chit-chat in Hebrew, and I think I did rather well.

I'd better get some sleep; it's almost 2 and I have a class at 8:30.

Goodnight!

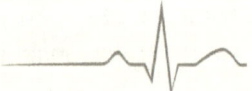

October 28, 2002, 12:45 a.m.

I've finally unpacked one of my large bags and I'm settling into my new place. Tomorrow morning, I'm going to a leadership seminar through MDA. Yael will be there, and Adee. It should be fun, interesting, etc. It's at Kiryat Moriah, where we had our course this summer, and I get free food and lodging. Next week, our Talmud class is going to the Dead Sea for a spiritual retreat. Sounds right up my alley: art, music, movement, learning. I'm excited.

I'm having a great time at Pardes; it's a truly stimulating learning environment in which I'm beginning to feel quite comfortable. Learning in *chevruta* differs greatly from any type of learning I've ever done; it reminds me of when my high school friend Bianca and I used to sit on my bed and quiz each other before exams. In *chevruta*, you and your partner help each other sift through the text. It's not only in Hebrew (which would be a breeze for me) but mostly in Aramaic, which makes it quite onerous. However, I am fascinated by the way the rabbis worked, by their thought processes and the arguments they bring up. I have been learning with Chaim, one of my housemates. We work pretty well together, so it's good. In my Modern Jewish Thought class, I've had various partners; today I was with Shalom, a twenty-six-year-old engineer from Seattle who is starting the army in December. There are really interesting people at Pardes, from unique backgrounds. Since I'm a people person, I love getting to know everyone.

There was another suicide bombing today, the second in a week's time. This one was at a gas station/restaurant in Ariel, a *Yishuv* in Judea and Samaria, an area also known as "the Shtachim," on the West Bank of the Jordan River. I believe that these places belong to my people, based on biblical history. However, I am not sure we should hang on to these places at the expense of lives. If it were true that we would have peace by moving our people out of Judea and Samaria, it might be worth looking into. But there is just too much hatred and extremism involved, sadly on both sides. Our neighbours won't be happy with our land; they want more than anything to "push us into the sea" and wipe out the Jewish presence in the Middle East. As sad as it sounds, it's true. It's an old hatred, but one that is very evident when living on this land.

I hope to start at MDA again on Wednesday; I first need an orientation at the station, and then begin riding the ambulances. I can't wait!

OK, I'm exhausted, enough writing.

Sleep tight, don't let any bedbugs bite. I'm sure they won't as I had a very restful night last night (albeit filled with one long crazy dream about love and finding my soulmate).

Lailah Tov.

October 30, 2002

I'm writing now from my apartment; at last we have a cable modem hooked up so I can write often. I'll now be able to respond to everyone who writes to me. I'm having the best time here. I just watched *Mr. Deeds* with my housemates; they're so great, and we all get along well.

Chaim is wonderful. He's a tall, blonde, teddy bear of a guy, from Florida. He feels like a big brother, and is quickly becoming one of my closest friends here. His kindness, joie de vivre and carefree open spirit make my life here joyful. I decorated my room today with all my pictures, and I finally feel at home. Being able to make a life for myself here is fantastic; I feel strong, happy, and settled.

Tomorrow I'm going with Yael to Tel Aviv to do some PR for MDA; we're meeting with a group from Colorado and we're supposed to tell them about our experiences at MDA. No problem! I have excellent things to say, of course. When I get back, I hope to be on time to hear a great lecture at Pardes on this week's Torah portion; it's *Chayei Sara*, my Bat Mitzvah portion. This even falls on the same day I read it, many years ago, in synagogue: November 2.

Today I gave blood. It felt wonderful, I suppose because of where I am; it felt spiritual, like I am really giving of myself to help Israelis. Tomorrow, Friday, I'm going to Beit Shemesh and will stay through Saturday night for Shabbat, with Manya and her family. I am looking forward to it, since I have never been there. I'll let you all know how it goes.

Anyway, I'm off to bed.

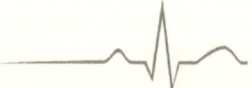

November 2, 2002

Just got back from a very relaxing Shabbat in Beit Shemesh with Manya's son Simcha, his sweet wife Merav, and their two little girls; Achinoam is three-and-a-half years old and Daniella is eight months old. I had a fun time playing with the kids, and the baby especially loved me (after her first initial crying fit).

It feels like all you do on Shabbat in Israel is eat and sleep, eat and sleep. Big Shabbat dinner on Friday night, a zillion courses; then Saturday morning you get up and eat cakes and do *kiddush* when the guys get home from *shul*. An hour or so later, you eat lunch, again an enormous meal of *cholent* (rice, barley, potatoes, meat all cooked in one pot). Then a few hours later, *Seudat Shlishit*, a "light" meal of challah, salads, kugel and more. Then later is dinner. And in between meals, you sleep, so I'm well rested.

It was wonderful seeing Simcha again, so long (ten years) after last seeing him. When I first met him, he was this cool guy in the Israeli army; he was my hero for a couple of years. Now he's got two kids, and they're the nicest family. It's great seeing people again that I haven't seen in so long.

Anyway, off to have a drink.

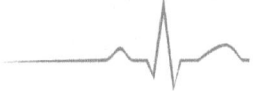

15

MDA Jerusalem - Day One

November 4, 2002

Shalom!

And now, the email you've all been waiting for...my first day at Magen David Adom Jerusalem!I was really nervous leading up to today because of the difficult time I had at MDA Haifa during the first week. Well, you'll be pleased to find out that today was *MEULEH*! I woke up at 5:30 and caught the 6:10 bus to MDA. The people there were really welcoming and helpful, and even though I only started at 9 (they have one driver who starts at 9 instead of 7; the same thing happened my first day in Haifa), my day was still amazing.

First of all, the volunteer I worked with was originally from the US and anglophone, so he helped me get adjusted without the language issues. My driver, Dudu, spoke really great English as well, so we spent the day alternating between Hebrew and English. Not that tall, but fit, bald and handsome, Dudu reminds me of that actor who played Imhotep in *The Mummy* (Arnold Vosloo). In fact, it was hard to get that reference out of my head, and slightly unsettling.

During our shift, Dudu was really patient with me and he's the first really good ambulance medic I've seen here so far. He took an EMT course at Humber College in Toronto (I applied there for paramedic school) a few years ago, and you can tell in the way he pays attention to detail. He takes time at the scene to do a good assessment, and today he even put a splint on a fractured leg (unheard of during my time at MDA Haifa, where in my experience they just bundle you into the ambulance and off you go, in agony). His skills and temperament really impressed me (cool, calm, fun to be with), and he made me feel safe and confident during our time together. As for my calls today... I had six!

The very first one was the most interesting; we were called to *Machsom Aram*, a military checkpoint. Apparently, we were quite close to Ramallah, just over the hill, I think. On the way there, we had to drive on the shoulder past a line of traffic that was blocked in both directions; there was a *hefetz hashud*. The police and military were present to ascertain if it was dangerous, and if necessary, to blow it up. We continued to the checkpoint where we waited for a few minutes for the army medics to bring us the patients - from the other side of the checkpoint. I've never seen a military checkpoint such as this except on TV; CNN etc, make the checkpoints sound horrific and inhumane, but to me it was just another border crossing. People walked across and showed their papers, and the soldiers mostly just glanced at them and let them pass. Each car was searched, and soldiers boarded each bus to check passengers. Honestly though, to me it looked like the traffic jams and checks performed by border guards at the US-Canadian border crossings such as Buffalo, Detroit, Cornwall... Not much difference, except more military khakis and bigger guns.

Back to the call: after some time, a military jeep drove up and told us we had to follow him through the checkpoint to the scene. Normally, the army medics bring the patients across to us, but not this time. They escorted our ambulance about one hundred metres past the checkpoint, to a terrible car crash between another military jeep and a car. There were three victims: two military police and one civilian. As per usual, at the scene of an emergency in this country, there was a huge crowd of people gathered. They were all Arabs or Palestinians, because that's the side of the checkpoint we were on. Soldiers kept the people back from the cars so we could work; we put one police officer on a backboard and put a cervical collar on the other one. We took them both in our ambulance while the civilian went in another ambulance.

That call was the perfect way to start my time at MDA Jerusalem, because I saw a totally different world than what I encountered in Haifa. Military, slightly dangerous, intense; but wonderful all at once. I don't quite understand what I'm feeling; I suppose some sort of adrenaline rush mixed with my love for Israel and my pride at taking care of her soldiers. I love how I feel, and I can't wait to continue experiencing these emotions.

My first day at MDA was filled with new experiences, new places, new people, new feelings. But most of all, it was filled with laughter, and camaraderie (can't say friendship yet, because I just met these people) and surprise. I had expected to have to put back up the shell I built this summer to fend off pain and sadness, and that I would have to fight for a spot on a good ambulance. But it all worked out, and overall I had a very laid-back, sweet day.

Let me conclude here with a couple of random "only in Jerusalem" stories:

1) Driving on the ambulance I looked out my window to see a *Sherut* driver. He had a "no smoking" sign hanging on his rearview mirror, and on his dashboard were three packs of cigarettes. On top of that, he had a lit one in his mouth! Only in Jerusalem.

2) The buses here all have little garbage pails by the middle door. In Canada, people just throw their trash on the floor, but here I observed three people in the span of a ten-minute bus ride actually get up from their seats, no matter how far, and throw out their trash. Then they went to sit back down. To me, that is beautiful. In a land with so many issues, so much stress, people take time to care about the cleanliness of public places. Jerusalemites impress me more every day.

I love this city. I fall more in love with Jerusalem and her fantastic array of wonderful people every day. The diversity of colours, clothing, religions, backgrounds, languages, and more is beautiful. My heart is full now, and complete; inside I feel a warmth that I know is satisfaction. It is surreal to me that in a country so heartbroken by war, so many hearts beat so strongly and vibrantly. You would think that the pain and stress inherent here would take a nice person and turn them hard, bitter, scared. But no — on the contrary. A smile here is easy to achieve — look at a girl on the bus who seems sullen and withdrawn, give her the slightest smile and a light turns on in her cheeks as she smiles back.

These tormented, tortured souls are reaching out to each other and to me, perhaps in order to transcend the pain. Here the agony seems to get channelled into *chesed*.

Maybe I'm an idealist, a romantic — of course, I am. But there is so much truth in what I just stated; I wish you could all feel the way I feel now.

I have never felt more alive.

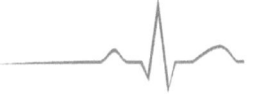

16

Filling the Spirit

November 6, 2002

Shalom!

I'm leaving Jerusalem for a few days; off to Kibbutz Almog, by the Dead Sea, for a "spiritual retreat" with Pardes. It should be nice and relaxing, just what I need after a bit of a stressful day yesterday. Here's what happened:

We were all sitting in the *Beit Midrash* at Pardes, learning in our *chevrutas*. We heard some rumbling outside; at first it sounded like thunder. Then came two loud sounds like explosions, and I was out of my chair in a flash, calling MDA people to find out if there was a bombing. Thankfully, that wasn't the case. So I went back to learning. Suddenly, a huge explosion/thunderclap type of sound hit us — the entire building shook and people in the room either dove for the floor or jumped out of their seats. Silence ensued, and looking out the windows, you could see shoppers, merchants, etc., coming outside to see what happened. I was sure it was a bomb; it felt and sounded exactly like what I expect a bombing to be. Thankfully again, that wasn't it. Turns out we'd been hearing airplanes, and one must have broken the sound barrier right above our heads — we heard and felt the sonic boom. This comes only two days after we watched an F-16 fighter jet circling the sky over Jerusalem. Needless to say, I was freaked out the rest of the day.

So I'm looking forward to a peaceful retreat, and soaking up some precious sun and warmth before winter comes and chills me to the bone (yes, it gets cold and damp here).

I miss you all, and I'll write when I get back on Friday.

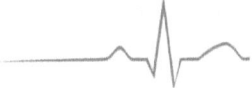

November 7, 2002: Kibbutz Almog

Pre-dawn at Kibbutz Almog, near the Dead Sea.

Gorgeous bright stars shine over my head among layers of white ephemeral cloud while birds begin to sing.

I star-watched at midnight and here I am again…

Brings me back to Pennsylvania forest peace — early morning with birds — last night I dreamt about birds landing on my shoulders and fluttering by my face.

A beautiful spiritual moment on this spiritual retreat.

Tomorrow I'm going to Tekoa for Shabbat with good friends. Should be nice, maybe difficult, and of course the ride up will be scary. But I hope I will take meaning from the experience.

Do I tell Mom and Dad before, or only after, I get back to Jerusalem?

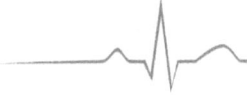

November 10, 2002, 12:10 a.m.

Shalom all!

I had a fantastic Shabbat with my friends in Tekoa. I have known this wonderful family since I was eleven and studying for my Bat Mitzvah; Barbara, the matriarch, taught me to chant the Torah and *Haftarah* in synagogue. I spent a lot of time during those years at her home, getting to know the whole family (four daughters, her musician husband Reuven and Barbara herself). They moved to Israel a few years later, and now live in Tekoa. Tekoa is a *Yishuv* in Judea and Samaria; it's about ten minutes past Efrat, if you know where that is. To get there, I had to take a bulletproof bus from Jerusalem; that was certainly an "adventure" for me. Taking the bus to the *Shtachim* is a completely new cultural experience, especially before Shabbat. There are only two buses every Friday from Jerusalem to Tekoa, so if you don't want to *tremp* you have to be on time. I caught the 2:20 bus after stopping to buy fresh flowers for my hosts and joined an eclectic mix of people heading out to the disputed *Shtachim*.

The bus itself is very safe; it's even hard to see out the windows because there are two layers of glass and the inner one is almost opaque. They were still transparent enough to allow me to watch as we drove through Arab villages and passed signs pointing the way to Ramallah, Beit Lechem, Beit Jala, etc. But I could also see the stunning scenery: desert hills speckled here and there with shrubs, wilderness, except for all the villages.

Upon arriving in Tekoa, I walked down to my friends' house, at the bottom of a hill looking out over a breathtaking view of desert and Arab villages. Honestly, an exquisite site. Tekoa has been growing steadily since its modern establishment in 1975; it lies on the ancient biblical site by the same name. Tekoa is where the prophet Amos was born, in the eighth century BCE. I really felt history around me, and I felt Israel around me.

We went to shul for Shabbat services Friday night, and I realized how much I love being in a small town where everyone goes to the same *shul* and knows each other: a real community.

What made this Shabbat even more special to me were the people I met; particularly two children. Keren is your typical fourteen-year-old girl, except for the somewhat haunted look in her eyes and the yearning for affection that emanates from her soul. I found myself sitting alone with her today for a few minutes, and she turned to me and said "I miss my brother." I asked her where he was, and when she said America, I asked her why he didn't come here to be with her. She said, "I think it's because he's traumatized by what happened — he's in and out of rehab... he's a druggie." I kept my mouth shut, knowing that if she wanted to confide in me, she would go on. Which she did. She continued to tell me, candidly, how her brother was in a car with her mother, father and a girlfriend, driving near Efrat. The car was attacked and shot at; her brother sustained arm injuries, her father who was driving was also injured, and the girl and Keren's mother were both killed. They were murdered. Keren sat across from me and just straight out told me this horrific incident in her life; I was stunned. It is really healthy for her to be able to talk about her pain; but such tragedy for such a young soul to deal with! I just wanted to fold her in my arms and stroke her hair, give her any type of contact and affection, but of course such action is probably contrary to what she needs. It's been a year and a half since Keren's mother was killed, and her father is about to remarry. I hope she heals and has as much happiness as possible for the rest of her life. She wears a bracelet with her mother's name, just as I wear one with the name of another terror victim.

Another visitor to the house was the young brother of one of the boys killed in a cave outside of Tekoa last year. Those two boys, Koby Mandell (thirteen) and Yosef Ishran (fourteen) went for a hike outside their *Yishuv*, and were ambushed by a group of Palestinians who bludgeoned them to death with rocks and their bare hands, leaving the cave where they were ruthlessly killed, splattered with blood. Such a horrific scene; such a horrific death. The families of these boys still live in Tekoa. The boy who came over on Shabbat seemed okay, yet he must be in so much pain each day.

They call these children *Nifgaei Terror*: victims of terror, or for a more precise translation, those hurt by terror. There is a fantastic support system for them in Israel, as there must be. But an invisible yet tangible veil hangs before their eyes; they have so much pain inside that lies so close to the surface that I could almost see it.

Yet, what can one do?

My Shabbat was extra special for bringing these children and their stories into my life. What to do with these stories? All I can do is pass them on to you, and hope you will pass them on to people you know, just so that these children and those they loved will not be forgotten in our daily existence. Keep at least one thought for the *Nifgaei Terror* each day, and perhaps somehow we can help them heal.

Let me tell you one more story of Tekoa, as I remember it, before I go to bed.

In Jewish law, a man must give his wife a *Get* when they get divorced, which is a legal document recognizing that they are no longer married. The *Get* allows a woman to go on with her life and re-marry if she wishes. Without a *Get*, a woman is forced to lead a lonely life because, according to Judaism, she is still married to the man she no longer sees as her husband. In Tekoa, there is a man who has refused his wife a *Get* for the past six years, and she no longer lives in Tekoa. The *Beit Din* has ordered him to give her a *Get* three times, and he still has not. The man must give the *Get* of his own will — they cannot force him or else the *Get* is not quite legal. Here is where the story gets interesting: the community got so sick of this man's cruelty that they decided to act. In synagogue one *Shabbat*, the reader interrupted the *Torah* service to read the prayer for the *Agunot* over and over. This prayer refers to the women who have not been given a *Get*. While he was reading the prayer, the women in the *shul* pushed aside the *mechitzah* and surrounded the man in question until he left the *shul*. He still hasn't given his wife a *Get*, but the people of Tekoa won't remain silent on the issue, I don't think. This story shows the power of community, and how Jewish law is applied in modern day society here in Israel.

I hope you've enjoyed your almost daily dose of Israel.

There's lots more to write, but it'll have to wait; I'm exhausted.

I miss all of you every day.

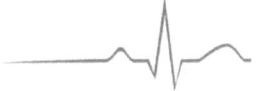

17

Eilat

November 11, 2002

Shalom,

Off to Eilat tomorrow for three days with Pardes. We're going for a five-hour hike at Ein Bokek tomorrow morning, and an eight-hour hike on Wednesday. I'm going to wear my feet out!!

I worked at MDA today — it was fun, especially when Yael hopped on my ambulance with a photographer from the *Jerusalem Post*. He took tons of pictures of me and another volunteer for an article this Friday on the overseas volunteers at MDA. So any of you here in Israel — pick up a copy of the Jerusalem Post this Friday.

Here's my funny story of the day: My ambulance was on a *nesiah dchufah*, lights flashing and sirens blaring. The drivers inevitably drive over sidewalks, on street dividers, going the wrong way down streets and into oncoming traffic. So today there were five of us (with the photographer and Yael included) and I was sitting on the bench in the back. The driver took a tight turn at speed and I went tumbling backwards off the bench, almost doing a back flip. In the process, I banged the back of my head on the rear door, and ended up sprawled on the patient bed (good thing there was no patient yet). Of course, I sat up with a big smile, laughing, when I really wanted to cry in pain — but at MDA you have to look and be strong, so that's what I did. You can see it, right? Sara falling backwards and looking like a clown, then popping up with a huge smile... We had a good laugh — always important on the ambulance.

Breaks any existing tension. I just hope the driver doesn't think I'm a klutz!

Miss you all.

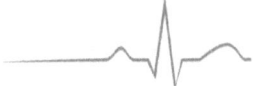

November 16, 2002

Shavua Tov!

I've had a very exciting week, culminating in a restful but disturbing Shabbat.

Let's begin with the *Jerusalem Post* article: Friday morning my phone didn't stop ringing, from 9 a.m. until *Shabbat* started around 4 p.m. Everyone had seen my picture in the *Jerusalem Post* — front page of the magazine section, and again inside it. Such a cool experience.

This week I spent three days in Eilat, at the southernmost tip of Israel on the Red Sea, on a *tiyul* with Pardes. We spent each day on a different hike, shlepping three or four litres of water on our backs because of the desert heat. The first day we spent in the Red Canyon, a spectacularly coloured area of the desert. The second day was the most exciting and the most strenuous. We climbed a mountain! Eight hundred eighty-seven metres of pain going up, and even longer coming down. Har Shlomo is a huge, black expanse of volcanic rock that soars upward from the desert to craggy heights of dry dusty magnificence. I was worried about my asthma, but I had no problems at all. We climbed up rock walls without ropes, using only our hands and feet and each other for support. I climbed between my friends Stu and Efraim, who helped me enormously; they got me over the psychological barriers of fear and lack of self-confidence. I was so proud of myself when we reached the peak — I never thought I could pull myself up a mountain, especially with a heavy pack and four litres of water on my back. I still can't believe I did it. Standing on that peak, I realized a dream that I never thought I would attain — to climb a mountain. I have always been fascinated by lofty heights and wished to reach them, but have always felt unable to do so. I proved myself wrong.

Although reaching the peak was incredible, what we witnessed a few minutes later cut my happiness and sent me spiralling into sorrow. We clambered down from the peak to a lower plateau to have a learning session. As we were beginning, we heard yelling from the ridge below the peak. I ran over to see a group of Israeli teenagers attacking an Ethiopian boy who was part of another group of hikers. A fight broke out between the white kids and the Ethiopians who were trying to just get away. The white kids were yelling things like *Kof Shachor* - black monkey. I couldn't believe my ears, or my eyes, that were watching kids throwing each other to the ground, punching and kicking each other and being egged on by their friends. Finally, the group of Ethiopians got away and started down the mountain. I had my gloves on and was ready to help injured kids, of which there were none, thankfully. I couldn't believe what I was seeing.

Once the kids had disappeared, a beautiful pregnant ibex walked through the same area that the kids had been fighting in moments before. She walked toward us, quietly and peacefully, and stopped for a few moments to look up at us. She was not scared, nor was she hesitant. I wonder if the fact that this ibex was pregnant is a sign that the future is pregnant with opportunity for change — and that we should work to change the status quo amongst our people. Sometimes it takes a striking and painful experience to force us into action. I hope I can find some way to incorporate this pain into something productive.

Back to the mountain — the way down was much more difficult than the climb up, with ropes, ladders, handholds in rock walls, and terrifying descents. In total, the hike took us about eight hours, and we found ourselves back on the bus around sunset.

The final, interesting part of the mountain climb was my chat with a classmate on the walk down. We hadn't yet talked, so he introduced himself and we talked for about half an hour as he told me his story. His fiancée was amongst those killed in the bombing at Hebrew University three months ago. His story was heartbreaking and almost too hard to bear, even as a listener. I admire him so much for still being here, and for trying to go on with his life. I don't know if I would be as strong.

The next day we climbed another mountain, called Har Hatzefachot. Later, we went rappelling down a sheer cliff wall, perhaps four stories high. It was scary!! Especially that initial drop over the edge, when you have to lean back in your harness and take the first few steps down the vertical wall. But once over the lip, I had fun bouncing down. At the end of the day, one of our group, who is a climbing instructor, came down the wall face-first, like the Navy SEALs do on TV. One woman decided she wanted to try, and she came down the same way. It was great until she reached the bottom and tried to stand up. Instead, she swung around and hit the wall with her head and cheek. I spent the next few hours taking care of her, helped by the Israeli army medic we had with us. Her face was covered in blood, which was streaming from the head wound and from some lacerations on her cheek. We cleaned her up, and I did a full assessment; luckily, she was OK. Just really in shock and scared. She was crying and shaky, and I spent quite a while just calming her down and reassuring her. She thanked me and went to a clinic when we got back to Jerusalem.

All in all, it was a very exciting trip. I surpassed so many of my psychological stumbling blocks and overcame fears such as heights and rock climbing. It was fantastic, and I feel like a new person. So alive!!!

Shabbat in Jerusalem only heightened that alive feeling — the joy of life here is most evident on Friday afternoons with the countdown to Shabbat. I spent my afternoon rushing around Machane Yehudah Market to buy veggies and fruit, challah and *rugelach* for my meal at my friend Shoshana's house (a friend from Pardes). At Marzipan (the best bakery in the *Shuk*) I ran into an old friend from Montreal, and we hung out while we shopped. It was great! *Shabbat* dinner at Shoshana's was great, although walking there was creepy because a vast tower of black smoke was rising from the area of the Old City. I still don't know what it was. Later in the evening, over dinner, I kept hearing explosions which freaked me out immensely. I found out today that there was a huge *pigua* in Hebron (about twenty-five minutes away) around dinner time — maybe I heard the bombings there — in which twelve soldiers and security men were killed and fourteen injured. Unreal.

Shabbat lunch was fantastic — I was invited to Aryeh's place, where he had all his cousins (about ten kids) over along with their parents. It was a fantastic meal full of speaking Hebrew and French; I felt at home.

Phew! Sorry for such a long email, but it's been an eventful week, as you can see. I am so happy here, even with the stress and heartbreak of *piguim*. I know I am supposed to be here — I feel that sense of destiny I felt this summer. My fate is wrapped up in that of my people; I honestly believe that. I know I will come back here after medical school and be a doctor here, helping my people. But I sense something else before that — what, I don't know. But I'm ready for whatever life and God want to drop in my lap.

I miss all of you and hope to hear from you soon.

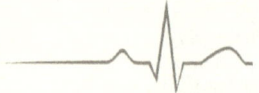

18

Pigua - Kiryat Menachem

November 21, 2002

Dear Friends and Family,

It's incredible how one phone call, one moment, can change your life. My phone rang this morning at 7:15; at first I thought it was my alarm going off too early. Scrambling to answer, I realized it was Aryeh on the other end of the line, telling me that there was an *Aran* underway. I got the location from him and jumped into my uniform, brushed teeth and ran out the door mumbling "shit, shit, shit." I sprinted to the street where a man stopped his car and offered to drive me to the site of the *pigua*. Turns out that bus #20 in Kiryat HaYovel had exploded at 7:14, the work of a suicide bomber. The man drove me halfway, then we hit a traffic jam, so I jumped out and ran down the street until I heard police sirens. I flagged them down and hopped in. They took me almost all the way to the incident before getting stuck in another traffic jam. So I again got out and ran, only to be picked up by a schoolteacher - she drove me to the street that was blocked off, and I ran the rest of the way in.

In the first car I jumped into, I prayed to God to help me get through this day; I said *Shema Yisrael* — the quintessential and most comforting Jewish prayer. I tried to gird myself for the scene to come. In the police car, the smell of burning set my respiratory tract on fire until I almost couldn't breathe; I'm not sure if that was the engine or if it came from the blown-up bus blocks away. I got to the scene at 7:30 and by then all the wounded had already been transported. As I ran in the last ambulances with victims were pulling out. There were still five or six ambulances there, with crews searching the park areas around and scanning the crowd for more wounded. As I walked in, I narrowly avoided stepping right into an immense pool of blood — but it just didn't hit me like it should have. For which I am glad, because I managed to keep functioning. Ahead of me I saw the wreckage of the bus; the same colour and type of bus I take all the time in Jerusalem these days. Sorry loved ones, but I need to get around here and the bus is the fastest, easiest way — but, of course, I avoid them as much as possible especially at rush hours, and walk most places.

Back to the scene: the *Pikud Eser* told me to stay with a certain ambulance, so I did. Suddenly, someone grabbed me and pulled me toward the crowd, where a lady had fainted. A medic was already there to help, and as I came up she was crying and moaning about her daughter, whom she thought was on the bus. I don't know if her daughter was killed, injured or never even there at all, but this poor lady broke my heart with her agony.

Back at the ambulance, I waited for instructions. It's not good to run around the bombing scene for many reasons (getting in the way, stepping on body parts, possibility of other bombs and shootings). Next to me was a police jeep, and all of a sudden I was swamped with young policemen needing their wounds cleaned. They had all cut their hands on the glass and pieces of the bus. People have interesting ways of coping with such situations; these guys were laughing and flirting with me, obviously to raise their spirits. So I went along with it. I think that's part of being a healer — even if you're dying inside, you need to help those around you cope as best they can. And their laughter helped me too.

As time went on, it became obvious that I didn't need to stay any longer, and the ambulance driver told me that if I wanted a lift back to the station, I needed to walk down to the bottom of the street and join the other MDA people. To do that I had to walk right past the bus and all the men cleaning up body parts and blood. The bus was a mess: burned, twisted steel, the windshield impacted as if someone had been thrown into it. Police were swarming it, collecting evidence and more. Hanging out the windows were MDA blankets, covering the bodies of the dead. I couldn't believe what I was seeing; and yet there it was. It was not a TV picture, although there were dozens of cameras right behind me as

I stared at the scene. It was not a bad dream, because I haven't woken up yet. It was real, it is real. Blood has a sticky-sweet smell.

I called Dad from that spot, while I looked at the pain sitting there in physical form before my eyes.

Continuing down the street, I met up with MDA and a few of my friends who worked at the *pigua*. A man was sweeping the street beside me, and I realized he was cleaning up any glass, bloody pieces of people, and anything else. In Judaism we must bury every part of a person, so this group called Zaka, made up of religious men, makes sure every bit is amassed after a bombing.

A few minutes later, a family approached me; the mother explained that her daughter and the daughter's friend needed to be transported to the hospital. I talked at length with them, two women about my age who were in serious emotional shock. The daughter had been about to get on the bus when she saw her friend coming down the street — so she waited for her instead. Then they saw the very same bus explode a few seconds later. Imagine that feeling — knowing you might be dead but for a quirk of fate, or God. They cried, and we put them in the ambulance. That's one wonderful thing about Israel and MDA — we take people to the hospital even if they're not physically but are emotionally hurt.

I got a lift back to the station with one of the ambulances. I hung out for two minutes with some friends there, but was really a wreck, so headed back to Pardes for some comfort. I decided to take the bus back because I knew that if I didn't get right back on the horse, I would never ride again. It's about conquering the fear they instill in you, and continuing to live in the face of intense anguish. So I rode home, lost in my thoughts and trying not to cry in my uniform. Must put on a brave-ish face. I was thinking about the scene, and people who lost loved ones, and the essential evil of these attacks. I was getting lost in pain with no clear light to help me. Sitting across from me were a young mother and her toddler; he began to cry and the soldier standing by them assisted the mother by giving her the baby's bottle that was on the floor. He smiled, and the baby smiled. And they smiled at me. That moment was like seeing the ibex on the mountain in Eilat, after that horrible fight. That moment gave me back my *emunah*, faith, and *tikvah*, hope that life will improve and that our people and its nation will survive. We will get through this. We have each other, and that's what's important.

Getting back to Pardes was a relief. I broke down and cried, but all my friends were there to help. I got amazing hugs, shoulders to lean on, tea and cookies, and incredible support. Afterwards I went home and Chen came over for lunch. I don't know what I'd do without her (thanks Chennie, I love you).

Then I went to Machane Yehudah Market and bought all the food I am now cooking for Shabbat. I needed to just throw myself back into Israeli society; it's like one big blanket to snuggle under when you're sad. Yes, people here can be hard to deal with, but they take care of you when you need it and they band together, sometimes, in the face of terror.

An event like today can shake or even break one's faith, but in my case it has done neither. Sure, I questioned and yelled at God often today, but that doesn't mean I don't believe He's there. And, now, I believe even more in the Jewish people, and in Israel.

I am hurting. I am in a lot of pain. But I am also thankful that I was able to help even in such a small way. My heart is broken, but I know it will heal again. Pain is a knife that cuts up your guts, but love and friendship are excellent sutures.

I miss you all. Just know that I am all right.

Pray for peace.

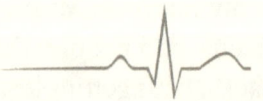

19

Chanukah and a Birth

November 28, 2002

Shalom!

I think it's been a little while since I last wrote. In fact, I believe the last words you all heard from me were pretty depressing. It's been an entire week since the *pigua* in Jerusalem, but there were three major *piguim* today as well. A shooting attack in Beit Shean, up north, left at least four dead and thirty injured. Two almost simultaneous attacks on Israelis in Mombasa, Kenya, left twelve dead and scores injured.

With all the violence, however, I have managed to have a pretty decent week. Until this week I have really been struggling with my learning at Pardes. I have felt very inadequate, almost stupid. Learning right now is not like learning in high school, when I was one of the "smartest" in my class. At Pardes, I am surrounded by incredibly intelligent and learned, dedicated and genuine people; they continually amaze me with their insight. We are studying Jewish texts such as the Talmud and the Gemarah, as well as Jewish thought and prayer. While I love the material and the discussion, I feel like a novice in a place full of experts. However, on Tuesday, I had a breakthrough, and the only difference in my day was that I got up for morning *davening* at 7 a.m. But, suddenly, all day long, I had incredible insights into what we were learning. I felt awake, alive, and smart again. Every class I developed new ideas and really felt the wheels turning... and the funny part of it all was that my prayer in the morning was completely static and unfulfilling, but it led to such intense understanding. I'm not sure how, but it's cool!!

I worked at MDA on Wednesday. I had tried to work on Monday, getting there at 6:30 a.m., but the ambulances were full and I had to go home. Since this is all volunteer work, and there are many volunteers, it occasionally happens that there is no space on an ambulance. On Wednesday, I worked with a great driver, an Arab Israeli guy named Halim. I don't know him very well, but he was kind and a good medic. We had five calls, which is a lot!

Our first call was a biker who had been hit by a motorcycle (not too serious) on the highway. What is a bicyclist doing on a highway? Your guess is as good as mine.

On the next call, we went into East Jerusalem to pick up a man at one of the clinics. We were told he had back pain. We arrived to a huge crowd of men and women, at least fifty, crowded around — just as any group of bystanders at an emergency situation — I suppose it's our ancient sense of bloodlust, "fascination with the grotesque" (phrase courtesy of my friend Liz). It was a bit of a dangerous scene, so Halim asked one of us to stay in the ambulance, doors locked, so it wouldn't get stolen. I was the first one out, wading through the crowd, and we found a man lying on the ground. Someone had hit him right in the back. We loaded him into the ambulance and took off.

Another time, we were called to the police station in the Old City to pick up a guy who had been in a scuffle with the military police. He was lying on the stairs, his face and head bloody, and he was complaining of excruciating pain in the lower right quadrant of his back. I think he was hit in the kidneys — that is a very painful place to be hit. We took him in the ambulance and I talked to him, cleaned his head wound, and we assessed him. He was not so stable, with an irregular pulse. He had a prior illness, blood in the lungs, so we wanted to get him to hospital right away. The gate was locked and the police wouldn't let us leave for a while. Finally, they insisted on putting one policeman in the back with us and one in the front seat of the ambulance. When we got to the hospital, they even handcuffed him, IV and all! I was not happy as the treating medic, but what do you say to big intimidating police? Especially since I didn't know the story — for all I know he may have tried to kill someone, or may have pulled out a bomb, or anything. I can't judge the police for their actions — the Israeli military is under *lachatz*, as we say here — and I have to trust them to be as fair as they can be in such a time of crisis as we live in now.

But that doesn't stop me from wishing someone had cared for my patient at the scene before we arrived, or from being angry at the policemen for cuffing his injured hands and legs together in the hospital bed.

Phew. OK, enough of that stuff.

It's CHANUKAH tomorrow! Lots of lights, olive oil, latkes, fun times with friends. For those of you who don't know, Chanukah is the Jewish holiday where we celebrate two miracles: the winning of the war against the Greeks, and a little pot of oil. The Greeks, under Antiochus, subjugated the Jews and forced many of us to convert. Men, women and children chose to martyr themselves rather than bow to Greek idols, and they were slaughtered. Jewish blood ran through the streets of Jerusalem, as it does almost cyclically throughout history, and does again today. We rose up against the Greeks and God made a miracle, pulling us through and allowing us to reclaim our religion. The Greeks desecrated our Holy Temple, but the Maccabees cleaned it up and found one little pot of oil, barely enough to light one lamp. But by a great miracle, that tiny drop of pure olive oil lit the *Menorah* for eight whole days.

We celebrate this holiday to remind ourselves God is always in the world with us and that even in the deepest darkness, He has given us little pots of oil that shine forth. We each have that little flame inside of us, and the Chanukah candles remind us to shine.

I went to the *shuk* and bought myself a little *Chanukiah* to light this holiday. I decided to light with olive oil this year, since I am in Jerusalem, instead of with wax candles. It will be an extra special, beautiful type of light.

I wish all of you a fulfilling Chanukah full of light, and I wish each of you (Jew and non-Jew alike) find strength to reach inside your souls and find that flame. Let it shine out through your eyes, your heart, your actions. Let all those around you feel its heat and rejoice in your brightly lit circle.

Open yourself to the knowledge that we can each make a difference in this world, if only we recognize the spark inside each of us as holy.

I miss all of you so much.

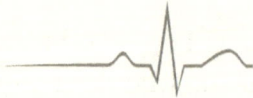

December 6, 2002

Shabbat Shalom,

I've had a wonderful Chanukah week, full of relaxation and work at MDA. There's so much to tell, I don't know where to begin. Each night this week I've been at a different Chanukah dinner or party. I am more tired today than when I'm at school all week long. Having Chanukah here in Israel, in Jerusalem, is so completely different from Canada. This is my first Chanukah without snow; it's been so warm the past two days I've been walking around in a T-shirt. I'm not sure I like Chanukah without snow. I've been very homesick and lonely, wishing I was with my family. I miss all of you.

Chanukah here is special because wherever you go there are *Chanukiot* burning brightly in the windows. I came home last night from MDA right at candle-lighting time (*shkiah*: that moment between sunset and darkness, when it's so beautiful that you could wear the air like a wedding dress). In the window above ours, and in the window above that one, were two families lighting their candles. I watched the children light, and listened to two different tunes for the blessings, and I felt so lucky to be here. Where else in the world are the Jewish people so free as here, where we can light our candles for the world to see?

Monday, my first call at MDA was a twenty-year-old Orthodox girl giving birth for the first time. We helped her through some contractions and then loaded her into the ambulance; she wasn't crowning yet. At the hospital, my driver allowed me and the other medic to go upstairs and watch the birth. The doctors let us assist, and a beautiful baby girl was born! What a wonderful experience; I almost cried from happiness.

I worked three days this week because I've been having an amazing time at MDA. There is one driver I really get along well with, his name is Dudu (don't laugh, it's really a cute nickname in Hebrew no matter what its English connotations may be). He is the first driver I worked with here at MDA Jerusalem and has rapidly become my favourite. I now preferentially try to get myself placed on his ambulance every day. We work really well together, and he is a great medic. Most of the Israeli volunteers don't enjoy working with him, because he likes to do most of the treatment himself (including blood pressure and pulse). However, after working with him three times, Dudu started trusting me and now lets me do almost everything. I asked him to let me know if I do something wrong, so I can learn, but he says I've been doing everything right so far. A couple of funny things about Dudu: being bald, he always smells of the sunscreen he rubs on his head, and for some reason he really loves to use polysporin for everything.

When I work with Dudu, it feels like I'm working with a real partner. This is what I imagine working as a paramedic in Canada would have been like if I had continued on that path instead of coming back to Israel this year. Dudu always stops at the best food places in the city and surrounding areas; some days we get shakshuka for breakfast, sometimes we stop at the yummiest falafel stands. We often go to a delicious restaurant, where they put a whole chicken schnitzel in a pita with salads, pickles, and french fries — the most filling and delicious lunch around. Another treat is when we stop for potato burekas filled with hard-boiled eggs and zaatar — scrumptious. Working with Dudu affords me the opportunity to sample all the gourmet offerings this city has!

We had some crazy calls this week — once we picked up an appendicitis case: a young female border police officer from the *Magav* base in Jerusalem. She was in a lot of pain and I hope she's already in the operating room.

My most interesting case by far (besides the birth) was on Wednesday. I was working with Dudu, and we got a call at 3 p.m. to a shooting. Dudu made the teenage volunteers get off the ambulance and stay at the station, so it was just me and him in the ambulance. Dudu made me put on a bulletproof vest; that was a pretty unnerving experience. Once we got to the scene, we found out that the gun was only shot into the air, so no one was actually injured. We took an Arab man who had allegedly been beaten by a plainclothes policeman. I'm not sure exactly what the story was, but the patient apparently had a long criminal record. Dudu started talking to him about the incident as we were driving to the hospital, and our patient got furious and agitated. Later I told Dudu never to do that to me again: I was sitting in the back with an agitated, dangerous man while Dudu was riding in the front. I had kept the vest on, but it wouldn't have really helped me, being so close to the man. Dudu apologized later, but wow did that ride allow me to feel the "fight or flight" response!

I went to the *shuk* today — it was fantastic as usual. Riding the bus just got much cheaper for me because when I paid for my *kartissiya* yesterday, the driver gave me a youth one instead of an adult pass. He saved me fifty shekels. For the same price as the adult pass, I now have double the rides. I really don't mind that everyone in Israel thinks I'm seventeen; I love feeling younger than I am.

OK, I have to go cook for Shabbat.

I miss all of you. Have a great weekend.

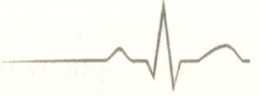

20

Love In, Love Out

<u>December 17, 2002   12:40 a.m.</u>

I'm having some wonderful days...

Last Wednesday, as I was walking home from MDA, my built-up, intense feelings of loneliness overpowered me. The sky was dark and stormy, and inside, my heart sent shivers of pain radiating up and down my limbs. I prayed to *Hashem* to send me my *Beshert*, or at least a guy to fill my heart and life for a while. I was feeling so alone, so unsatisfied, even in the most wonderful city in the world. Guilt washed over me as I realized how blessed I am: a loving family, close friends, a new *chevrah*, learning in Jerusalem, working at MDA... how could life be any better? God has given me everything I've ever wanted... and all I am missing, it seems, is love.

Thursday changed those feelings. There's a guy I study with at Pardes, named Dov, who is from the US. I think he's really cute, sweet and interesting; I guess I have a small crush on him. Dov and I went out for lunch after having a nice talk over hot chocolate. I think that our getting to know each other brought a lot of joy into our lives. I asked him if he wanted to get lunch with me, and he agreed. Later, after *Minchah*, I asked if we were going for burgers or pizza; he laughed and said, "I thought we'd go to Olive." Liz piped in, "You're taking Sara to Olive?? That's a date!" and he didn't deny it.

We left and walked down Emek Refaim Street to a beautiful little restaurant behind a pretty fence, and we ate outside under the open sky and trees. Leaves fell in my food, and even that felt holy. When the menus came, he asked if I wanted wine; of course I did! So over wine for me and Guinness for him, with a roast beef sandwich for each of us, we talked for two hours. When the bill came, I asked how much I owed, and he said, "I thought I'd pay it all." I chipped in a bit, but he wanted to pay the whole thing; I couldn't believe it. That's got to count as a date, but I'm trying to stay grounded, as my friends have advised.

After lunch, we went fruit shopping, and we each bought two mangos and a melon. When we finally parted ways, he gave me a great, lingering hug. We made plans for me to cook him dinner one night, for us to see *Lord of the Rings 2* with a couple of other people, and for him to come over and watch *Scrubs* episodes with me. It was a wonderful day.

Today he and I went grocery shopping together after community lunch at Pardes. We spent a good hour in the store and had a fun time. On our way out, he spotted a *shuk* rigged up in the side alley and asked if I wanted to go; so we went. I love how spontaneous he is. He admired all the fabrics from India, especially these beautiful fans that are meant to hang on your wall. He actually bought one, painted with elephants bathing in a river. We also bought some little toys that I previously bought this summer in Haifa; the ones that are like slinkies, that bounce and are on key chains. We had a really glorious afternoon together, and again when we left each other, we had a nice hug. He invited me to watch a movie tonight with a few other people, but he never called, so I figured he fell asleep or forgot. That doesn't bother me; we're grown-ups, right? If he wants to see me, he'll make the effort. After all, today he skipped class to go shopping with me; he's the one who asked me if he could come along. So I feel pretty confident that he enjoys being with me.

I feel like my fervent prayers of last week were answered. This is a man that I can truly see myself with. I'm trying to keep my feet on the ground and not expect much, but I can envision a strong future with Dov.

I'm going to bed now - long day tomorrow culminating in two football games. Dov is the quarterback for one of our Pardes teams, and I make it a point to go watch them play.

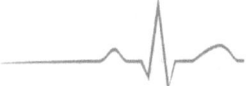

December 21, 2002 - Winter Solstice

What a difference one week makes… last Shabbat I spent thankful for a wonderful guy entering my life, finally. This Shabbat started out sweet, at Yakar (a small, cozy *shul*), with very meaningful *davening*, but swiftly deteriorated into tears. Things with Dov are over; he hurt me so intensely Friday night at dinner that I can't even think of being his friend. I don't want to discuss it more than that, but I walked home at 12:30 a.m. on my own, with the wind in my face, crying. I cried until 3 a.m. and went to bed.

Moving on, I want to write about a couple of moments in my week that stand out….

While riding the ambulance with Dudu on Wednesday, a white dove flew at us out of nowhere. She flew directly at the ambulance; thankfully, Dudu has incredible reflexes and managed to avoid killing her. What would possess this bird that she should come at us kamikaze-style? Why would the bird of peace fly a suicidal mission? How metaphorical this dove seems to me. Peace hurling herself at us, not realizing in her desperation to connect with us that she may kill herself in the process.

Shabbat evening, Chaim, Liz and I walked to our friend Miriam's for dinner. On the way, a tremendous crash sounded all around us. Hoping beyond hope it was not a bomb, I steeled myself. Within a minute or two, lightning lit up the Shabbat night, and we knew the storm was building to a climax. While crossing Derech Hevron (the road we were on) we said the prayers for hearing thunder and seeing lightning. The moment after Chaim said Amen, a gigantic bolt of lightning ripped the sky. An enormous clap of thunder followed, and within a few seconds hail accosted us as we hurried to shelter. It was remarkable how quickly God seemed to respond to my prayers of gratitude; almost as if He was demonstrating how powerful His works truly are. The storm continued all night, soaking us each time we left one place and moved to the next. What a beautiful show of *Hashem's* strength; what a special feeling to be in Yerushalayim in a hailstorm.

I'm going to bed, *lailah tov*.

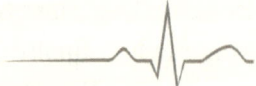

December 24, 2002   12:43 a.m.

Spent today at MDA, working with a driver named Hellman (yes, like the mayonnaise). It was a fun day with a few interesting calls. An important Jewish lawyer, a very high-ranking officer, got roughed up by soldiers at the checkpoint near Beit Lechem. Apparently, he was trying to pass some papers to someone on the other side of the checkpoint. I'm not sure what the exact story is, so I can't judge anything. His nose was broken in the scuffle and he was very upset. I felt awful for him, for the pain and confusion he felt at being hurt by the military, but he must have done something very suspicious to have been treated as he was.

Had a long day with Dov yesterday, at the MDA course. I tried to ignore him and be aloof all morning, but at our first break, he followed me outside and asked me why I was so sad. I didn't tell him, I only told him that I'd been having a rough couple of days. He gave me a hug, and broke all my defences. I'm pathetic, huh? I just want to write down one of our conversations yesterday, that will play over and over in my head for a while.

Dov: "You're a really great schmoozing person. I love hanging out with you."

Sara: "Thanks, I enjoy being with you too."

Dov: "I can't wait till we get to medical school together, and we can study and hang out all the time."

Sara: "Me too."

Dov: "Then later on we'll open a practice together!"

Sara: "Sure." Then a brief conversation about subjects to specialize in.

Then Dov talked a bit about his aunt, who has two adorable little kids. He talked about how he wants children soon. I told him I also want kids, by the time I'm thirty.

Sara: "When I finish med school, I want to make *Aliyah* and live on a *moshav* with my husband and kids."

Dov: "I also want to live on a *moshav* one day."

Sara: "Uh-huh."

Dov: "We're going to spend our whole lives together! We're never going to get rid of each other!! I'm never going to get rid of you!" (Sarcastically at the end.)

Sara: "I'm never going to be rid of you! Scary thought!"

— awkward silence —

Dov: "So, did you come to Israel to find your *Beshert*?"

Sara: (shocked) "Yeah, I guess I did."

Dov: "Me too."

Sara: "I felt my destiny calling me here this year, of all years. I don't know why."

Dov: "I felt the same thing."

Then we had to go back inside.

Crazy, no? But I get the feeling I'm not the kind of girl he wants to be with right now; rather, I could be his "final woman," as I told Liz. He's someone I could end up with.

I want him now, though.

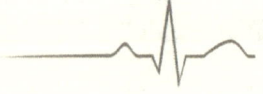

21
Dichotomy of Home

December 30, 2002

Shalom everyone,

It's been such a long time since I last wrote that I can't even remember what I wrote about!

Life here in Jerusalem has been relatively quiet recently, thankfully, and my life has taken on a semblance of normalcy. I study three days each week, volunteer at MDA twice a week, and rest on Friday and Saturday. "Rest" — the quote marks are key — because every Friday night someone has a nice big dinner and Saturday someone else has a nice big lunch. Shabbat in Jerusalem is a day to be with friends, eat, sing and be happy. I love it, but I am always more tired after the weekend.

Great news; I have one med school interview scheduled already — March 3 at New York Medical College. Hopefully, I can schedule the other NY med school interviews over that one week.

What do you think? Should I come home for my birthday, or celebrate it here in Jerusalem?

I finally got my passport back the other day, with my temporary residency permit for Israel! I was so excited to see it; a permanent record and proof that I really am living in Israel this year. It's hard to express how wonderful I feel seeing the permit in my passport. Whenever I look at it, I am reminded I took a drastic step in my life that turned out to be the exact right thing to do.

More and more I realize what an important year this is for me. I am growing each moment; my spiritual development is very high right now. I am immersed in a culture that surrounds me like a pillow. As hard as it is sometimes to live with Israelis (subtlety just isn't a known concept here), the rewards are indescribable. Let me try to explain using examples:

Twice each week I ride the #7 bus to and from Magen David Adom. The drivers recognize me now. Last week I rode home with one driver who asked me how my day went, and I told him how tired I was. Today I ran and caught the bus home with the same driver, who remembered our conversation from last week and asked if I was tired again today. In Montreal, I rode the buses to and from school for five years of high school, and not once did I have a personal conversation with a driver.

Wearing my Magen David Adom jacket around Jerusalem is an intense experience; it singles me out as an individual who is actively involved in helping her people. I become as visible as a soldier, or a police officer; each of our professions is equally respected and appreciated by the people of Israel. In Canada, ambulance workers are respected, but nowhere near the way they are here. Israelis know that those of us wearing the MDA uniform are there on the front lines. Israelis know that each MDA worker or volunteer is prepared to jump in to help in any crisis. We are treated so well here, and I feel truly loved in this country. I am so happy to be able to give to my people in this special way; all my life I have dreamt of using my skills to help the Jewish people and Israel.

Other news in my life: I helped teach an MDA course last week, and trained another entire crew of foreign volunteers who will be riding on ambulances starting next week. When one of my teachers at Pardes realized where I was last week, she asked me if I would teach her and a group of her friends how to perform child and infant resuscitation. Of course, I agreed right away. If I can help even one mother save her child in an emergency, I will have performed a great service.

I met a nice guy. No more to be said about it — it's probably just friendship. But it's nice to hope.

That said, it's time to sign off. Please write soon - I miss you all so much. Sometimes it's almost overwhelming, the sadness at being torn between two continents. I don't know if any of you know the music of Achinoam Nini (Noa) - she's a fantastic Israeli singer. There is one particular song of hers that expresses how I feel about Israel and Canada:

<u>Pines</u>

Lyrics: Leah Goldberg

English Translation and Music: Achinoam Nini (Noa)

Reprinted with permission from the artist

https://noasmusic.bandcamp.com/track/pines

Here I will never hear the blue-jay's song elated

Here a tree with twig of snow I will not find

But in the shade of all these solitary pines,

All my childhood is reincarnated.

The tingling of the needles is gone

Homeland I will call a snowy distant dream

Greenish frost and ice enclose a mountain stream

A stranger's land, a foreign tongue in song.

I remember those snow-capped mountains

And a song on F.M.93

Oh my darling, I have grown with you

But my roots are on both sides of the sea.

Perhaps only the migrating birds can ever know

As they're suspended between the heavens and the earth below

The pain I feel as I am torn

I have been planted and replanted with the pines,

And it is with them I have grown

But still my roots spread over the sea

In a dichotomy of home.

Goodnight, sleep tight.

Speak to you soon, I hope.

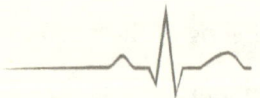

January 5, 2003

Dear Everyone,

Big double suicide bombing this evening in Tel Aviv.

Twenty-two dead, over one hundred injured.

I'm okay; being in Jerusalem, I was nowhere near the carnage.

Thank God.

I'm working at MDA tomorrow.

Pray for peace.

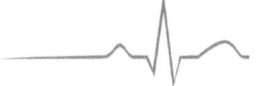

22

Waiting for War

January 9, 2003

Shalom everyone,

My emails have been quite sporadic lately, but to tell you the truth, it's because I have so much to say but I'm afraid to say it. I don't want to censor myself, especially at such a crucial time in my life. So let me preface this letter by saying it will be disturbing, and it will be frightening. Mom, Dad, considering our conversations about the impending situation here in Israel, you might not want to read this letter just yet. But please understand it is vital to tell the story as it unfolds, from my unique perspective here. I love you very much, but I also love this country and my people, and for their sake, I must tell my stories honestly.

I want to write about war. Israel is a scary place to be in right now, of course, but adding to the daily fear of terrorism is the imminent threat of war. Each day is filled with anxiety over when, where, how, what, and will we survive? Soon the US will attack Iraq, and we here in Israel will suffer the consequences. I remember being in grade six in 1991 during the Gulf War, and writing letters to Israeli schoolchildren to let them know we cared about them. I remember the news footage of children wearing gas masks, and I can vividly recall sitting in our classroom saying prayers for Israel. But then I also remember the incredible feeling we had when we realized the miracle: so many Scuds rained down on Israel, and hardly anyone was killed.

Now I am here, in Jerusalem, and perhaps a geeky, blonde Akiva School girl, with glasses and pimples and love in her heart, is sitting in her classroom writing letters to the children I met at synagogue last Friday night.

I walked by a bus shelter today and a gigantic sign was hanging inside: a picture (taken during the Gulf War?) of children studying in a classroom, with each one wearing a gas mask. At the bottom of the sign, in Hebrew, was written "It is coming in January." What a way to stir up mass hysteria! Quite irresponsible, in my opinion.

When we visited my friend Miriam tonight, we noticed that the window of the bomb shelter in her building was open. Glancing inside, one could see a dark, musty space. The heavy, bolted metal door had been opened, as we could see from tracks on the floor. Obviously, the building caretakers had begun to clean out and prepare the shelter.

Riding the ambulance on Monday, I noticed a new, locked, green kit: the chemical and biological warfare emergency response kit. Inside is ONE chem/bio warfare suit, as well as materials needed in the treatment of patients during such an event. The protocol at MDA is only two people on an ambulance responding to a *nefilah* (literally, falling; the dropping of chem/bio weapons on the populace).

Now, you're all wondering why I am here at this point; why haven't I come home? Next question: What am I doing to prepare myself for war? How will I be safe? Am I crazy?

I'm going to try and answer those questions...

Why am I still here?

Well, why did I come to Israel in the first place? To work on the ambulances and save lives, and to contribute in any way possible to the security and moral support of my people. I am here because I love this place, this country, this nation. I am staying because I love all the above. I cannot leave. Could you abandon a loved one in time of need? Obviously not — and as such, I cannot abandon a country full of loved ones in this terrible time of uncertainty. Add to that the fact that many of the MDA personnel will undoubtedly be called up for reserve duty, leaving a void that cannot be filled by the thousands of teenage volunteers (they are not allowed to go to these types of situations). Who will MDA rely on? I plan to be there to save lives.

What to do to prepare?

First, my gas mask will arrive shortly. My school is supplying each of us with a mask and extra filter, just as the rest of the Israeli population has. Next, my roommates and I are preparing a sealed room. Each dwelling in Israel must have one of these during war, for the occupants to hide, in case of chem/bio warfare. We will seal the one small window with plastic sheeting and packing tape, and once inside, we will seal the door similarly, with a wet towel stuffed in the crack with the floor. We're stocking the room now with a week's worth of water, dried food, canned food, first aid supplies, batteries and flashlights, radio, blankets, pillows, etc. The room we've chosen has internet access, phone jack, many outlets and a power bar, and only one little window. We will be OK. If I am at MDA during an attack, I will jump straight into a protective suit and head out in the ambulance. Otherwise, I will get into the sealed room with my gas mask on, and huddle tight with my roommates.

How will I be safe?

By using all the precautions delineated by the Israeli government and the military. These standards have improved a lot since the last Gulf War, and we know that hardly anyone died then (I think only two died from the direct impact of Scud missiles). I plan to be fine, of course.

Am I crazy?

I suppose that's the key question in your minds. For a straight answer: yes, I suppose I am slightly off my rocker, but in a good way. Being here, amongst my people, in Jerusalem, has done something to me that I never imagined. This place fills me up. Israel completes me. I have found eternity in each moment here. Yes, I am crazy; crazy about this land and her people. I'm involved in a love story that I only dreamed about as a child. I dance with the music of Jerusalem in my heart every night when I walk home under the stars. Above me, stars twinkle while ahead of me as I walk down the hill, the lights of Jerusalem twinkle as if in response to the call of the stars. Yesterday I was in the *Beit Midrash* at Pardes, and the colour of the sky stopped me in my tracks. The sky was golden — as golden as the dome atop the Temple Mount, golden as the ring on my pinky finger, golden like honey on Rosh Hashanah apples. In the middle of the sky hung the new moon, and below it the lights of Jerusalem shone in the same hue as the vivid sky above.

Yes, this is a frightening time to be in Israel. But it is also a most exhilarating experience. I am so alive here. I am more alive than I have ever been, and each moment of each day imbues me with a new spirit and joy for life. Love has blossomed in my heart; spirituality has rekindled itself in my soul. I am connected to each bird, each blade of grass, each drop of blood I encounter on the ambulance. Each hand I hold or shoulder I touch in comfort when I work for MDA lights another flame in my heart. How many of us can truly say we feel fulfilled? How many of us have felt true satisfaction from life? Are you as happy as I am? If you cannot answer this last question with a resounding "yes", then you must understand why I choose to be in Israel right now. Simply put: I am happy.

I miss you all. I love you.

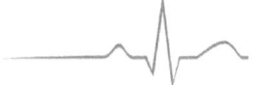

January 15, 2003

Hi everyone,

I'm going out of town in six hours; I will be back in Jerusalem on Saturday night.

We're heading out on a *tiyul* with Pardes, to Kibbutz Ketura in the Arava Valley (down south). It's been raining like crazy these past two days, so we're a bit worried about flash floods — that may nix our hiking plans.

It will be nice to get away for a few days.

Miss you all.

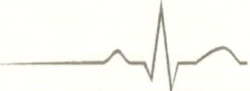

January 16, 2003   Sometime between 5-6 p.m.

On a rocky hill in the desert of the Arava.

We set off in the late afternoon, to a location in the wild desert. As a spiritual exercise, we were tasked with sitting alone in the open space as night fell around us. Our teachers asked us each to ponder how it felt to be alone in the desert, and to consider what characteristics of the desert made us feel that way.

I built a little rock shelter for my candle, and only after did I consider the possibility of a scorpion under those rocks. I sat there and, while I felt that sense of awe and contemplation that solitude in the desert engenders, I also found myself running over survival scenarios in my head. I felt conflicted — peaceful, yet anxious.

By staying still and quiet, I could hear the desert wind whispering to me. I felt safe, cozy and protected, nestled on the still warm ground by a small flame, but every now and then I remembered the dangers inherent in this place.

The desert outside is like the desert inside — scary, dry, fearful in those alone times. Yet all around the desert, life stirs, especially in the darkest hours. It is a miracle the chain of life flourishes here, just as the marvel of our own survival when often we feel lost.

And my candle flickered and hung on, barely, brightly, as the soul of the Jewish people clings always to existence. I built a shelter for my flame, just as we have we built a shelter for our nation here in *Eretz Yisrael*.

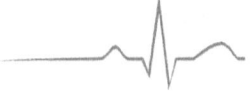

23

Gas Masks and Monsters

January 25, 2003

Hi everyone, *shavua tov*.

Things are going well here in Jerusalem. I can't believe I live here! That fact is still overwhelming.

I had a nice quiet Shabbat, ate meals with small groups of friends, and relaxed. I went to services at Shira Chadasha, an Orthodox congregation started a little over a year ago by one of my teachers and a group of her friends. This congregation is unique because it is Orthodox, but women are equal to men. There is still a separation between men and women, in the form of a sheer white *mechitzah* — but this *mechitzah* runs straight down the middle and you can see through it. Women lead *Kabbalat Shabbat*. Women also read Torah, at a table which is split down the middle by the *mechitzah*, so men and women pray together and read Torah together but still apart. It's a great balance, and one that I could see myself adopting in my synagogue life. The only problem is that the *Ruach*, or spirit of the service, was not what I am used to (from praying at a high-spirited and motivated service every Friday night that I've been here, called Yakar); but perhaps this week was out of the ordinary, and the spirit will be higher at other times.

In any case — it's been a great Shabbat.

I wanted to let you all know that I will be coming home for at least one medical school interview (I hope more!). I arrive on March 5 and leave a month later. So anyone who wants to see me before July or August should make sure they're in Montreal. Anyway, I have to run — I'm going to a concert tonight.

Have a great week!

January 29, 2003

Today I worked at MDA for the first time in a week. Last week I was sick with some sort of cough that I caught on our *tiyul* to Kibbutz Ketura, so I didn't work on Wednesday. Then this Monday we had a gas mask demonstration at Pardes, so of course I didn't miss that. Today was, therefore, quite refreshing; working at MDA always makes me feel energized (I suppose it's the result of adrenaline and passion).

Let me first write about Monday's demonstration. A soldier from the Home Front Command came in to educate us on what to do in the event of an attack. She gave us thorough information on the types of chemical and biological weapons that Iraq might deploy against Israel: nerve gas, mustard gas and anthrax. She clarified that the odds of Iraq managing to hit us with this stuff are very low, and even if Saddam manages to get his missiles past the Israeli air defences, they will land nowhere near Jerusalem (too many Muslim holy sites here). However, it is still important to know what to do in the event of an attack. We learned about when to go to the bomb shelters, how to make a sealed room and what to stock it with. She also told us the basic first aid for a mustard gas attack (cover the affected area with flour or baby powder, leave it on about thirty seconds till it turns yellow, and brush it off into the trash, repeat until the powder stays white). In the case of a nerve gas attack, we have an atropine syringe in the gas mask kits, to be used only if our area was affected and the media advises us as such. The atropine is the only proper treatment for nerve gas, and you inject your thigh just as you would with an epipen: jab the syringe into your leg and the needle self-injects. Once you've injected yourself, you bend the needle into a hook and attach it to your shirt collar so that your rescuers know you've taken it. Finally, we learned how to prepare and use the gas masks. Since I have asthma, I get a special mask with a battery-operated blower that works on positive pressure. It's supposedly easier to breathe in that mask... we'll see. We don't have our kits yet. The masks even have a straw for drinking.

The next day, election day, Ehud Ya'ari (famous Israeli journalist) came to speak at Pardes about the *matzav*. He offered his perspective on the Iraq crisis, elections and terrorism. It was very interesting to listen to him; he predicts the war will start around February 24.

I leave March 5 for Canada, and hopefully, medical school interviews. I'm getting nervous since I only have one so far (at New York Medical College) and I'm on the waiting list for one at Rush. I will be home for approximately one month. My parents want me to come home earlier to avoid the war, but I really want to be in Jerusalem for my birthday (when will I get this chance in the near future?).

Finally, we arrive at today, and my day at MDA. I worked in an outstation called Pisgat Ze'ev, in East Jerusalem, with a driver named Marilyn. We only had two calls all day, but they were both as sad as they were interesting. The first one was a twenty-eight-year-old woman in her ninth month of her third pregnancy. She fainted on the bus, and we took her to the hospital in distress. I hope her delivery went okay today.

The second call was one of the most distressing I've had to deal with. I have had other very hard, hellish calls. Some that come to mind are the *pigua*, major trauma in car accidents, a young mother who attempted suicide two weeks ago by overdosing on pills, a man who fell/jumped/was pushed from a roof in Haifa and his brains were on the sidewalk, a two-year-old boy who pulled a vat of boiling soup off the stove all over himself, etc. I could go on.

But today's call was painful for different, deeper, reasons...

We were taken by police escort to Beit Hanina, a Palestinian sector of Jerusalem, where we followed a car of men who took us to a residential building. We climbed the six flights of stairs to find a locked door and a woman screaming behind it. One man (a cousin of the patient) had keys and unlocked the door. Inside was a seventeen-year-old girl in the second month of pregnancy. She was hysterical, crying and screaming. In the other room lay the heavy black bat that her husband had beaten her with. It was obvious that he had obtained this weapon with the pure intention of hitting his wife with it. There was no other use for such a bat. It was hewn off at one end and covered in duct tape; the perfect length and size for a powerful man to handle as a club. Sick. Back to the girl: she was beaten all over her body, from head to feet. He had punched her repeatedly in the back and in the face, and hit her with the bat in the legs, arms, stomach... even pregnant. This was not the first time; apparently a similar incident had occurred last year, but the police did nothing to the husband. So the girl stopped calling the police, figuring that her husband's repeated beatings would just be shrugged off. This time, however, he didn't only beat her and kick her and step on her - he took her passport and her one-and-a-half-year-old daughter's passport, and dragged the child from the house. He ran off with her, and the police are out looking for them. Imagine this seventeen-year-old girl beaten badly and with her daughter kidnapped by an abusive man. What a horrific situation.

The girl only spoke Arabic and English, so I became the primary caregiver. In the apartment, I tried my hardest to calm her down, regulate her breathing, and prevent her from going into a deeper state of hysteria. When we finally got her to come outside with us, there was a group of men waiting, who laughed and pointed at her; these were her husband's friends. A bunch of sick, twisted animals, revelling in the pain of a woman. We took her in the ambulance and while the other medic took her blood pressure and pulse, I held her head in my hands and tried to keep her breathing slowly. I treated her like I would my sister, stroking her hair and cheek, reassuring her. She calmed down, and lay there quietly, crying.

Once at the hospital, we put her in a bed, and her aunt was there with her. I can't express how incredible a feeling it is to be able to communicate non-verbally with someone; her aunt only spoke Arabic, and she thanked me. I understood the intention behind her words, and the kiss she blew me from her seat by the bed. I connected with the look in her eyes, and I felt the emotion behind the hijab she wore. Those last few moments in the emergency room were so intensely beautiful, because I truly felt that connection between people that overrides any cultural, religious, ethnic or political walls we've constructed between us. Working for MDA is so incredibly amazing precisely because I walk into a scene wearing a red Magen David, the symbol of the Jewish People, but at the same time that Magen David etched into my soul burns brighter than any symbol. My *neshama* works through my hands when I put those latex gloves on. I can feel my innermost spark reaching toward every person I help. There is a link forged between souls when my gloved hand touches someone. With healing, I reach past concrete and steel walls to touch goodness on the other, hidden, side.

What I felt when I touched that girl today tore me up inside. I felt the agony of a child stuck in a cage she cannot escape, tormented by the animal of her nightmare world. I sensed the raging of a captured lioness, unable to free herself or strike back at her oppressor, and incapable of finding her stolen cub. How helpless she must have felt; her daughter in the hands of a sadist and her own body hijacked by his fists. There is only so much I can heal when I come to a scene. I never learned and will never know how to fix wounds of the soul.

She reminded me so much of my little sisters, and I wanted to take care of her like I take care of them when they cry and need my strength. I wanted to take her in my arms and rock her like a baby, stroke her hair and tell her, "everything is going to be all right." Unable to reach out to her like that, I settled for stroking her hair and cheek, holding her hand, and making sure she knew I was there and taking care of her.

Why do people do such things to each other? How can a man take a club to his beautiful young wife, who is feeding his first child outside and his second child within? Did the police find him, is the child all right, will he be punished? Will she go back to him when the bruises fade and her humiliation is but a memory? Did she lose the baby?

Today was a hard day, but also filled with sunshine. The rain only started when my shift ended. The wind woke me up this morning even before my alarm, and stepping outside, I was greeted by a sliver of crescent moon and one bright star hanging over Jerusalem. Perhaps the rain can wash away some of the pain shed on the streets of this city. Perhaps the blowing wind can cool the scrapes on the knees of a hurting nation. This weekend is *Rosh Chodesh*, the new moon, the new month. The month of Adar, the month of joy in our Jewish calendar; the first day of which is my Hebrew birthday. On Sunday, I will be twenty-four years old. I will celebrate my birthday. I will sing with joy at being here, in Jerusalem, in Israel, with my people and our cousins and extended family. Sure, we try to kill each other, and there is hatred and destruction and murder, but I cannot stop it myself. I cannot continue to work as a healer and at the same time take in all the pain. I must feel that agony and understand it, but not absorb it. I must touch it, grasp it, examine it and recognize it; but then I must brush it off my skin like mustard gas. But instead of putting it all in the trash, I have immortalized it here on these pages. You know what it is; you know that I have felt it and will feel it again. You are all my witnesses. If one day I am heartless or cruel, place these words before me and remind me of my own testimony. In such a way, I can help this girl today and others I will encounter in the future. My healing skills are not good enough to help them any more than that.

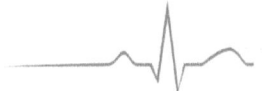

24

Land of Cats, Doves and Nightmares

February 3, 2003

Shalom all,

Just got back from a quiet, boring day at MDA. It's a good thing it was quiet today, because Saturday night I spent an hour in the emergency clinic getting an asthma treatment. My lungs aren't taking very well to the fact that the Jerusalem weather has changed drastically in the span of a couple of days — today we've got a sandstorm, and asthmatics, old people and kids were warned to stay inside. Oh well, what can you do? That's life in a desert land.

I spent my Shabbat in Tekoa with Barbara and her family. I had a fantastic time. The bus ride out there on Friday afternoon was not the best. As it was the last bus before Shabbat, it was packed, and I had to stand with a dozen other people in the cramped aisle. The bulletproof buses have minimal space inside, so you can imagine how cramped it was. As we came closer to the outskirts of Beit Lechem, the driver told us everyone standing had to sit on the floor for the next five minutes. This is because the top of the bus, between the windows and the roof, is not bulletproof — and people standing in the aisle naturally would make good targets. It was the strangest feeling, to sit on the floor of a dark bus with all the other Jews trying to get somewhere before Shabbat. The thoughts that went through my head were intense. I asked myself why it should be such a familiar feeling to me, as a Jew, to sit in a cramped dark space and pray for peace around me? My thoughts wandered to the Jews during the Holocaust, crammed into cattle cars, then to the Jews on the Exodus ship who squeezed their way toward hopeful freedom in our homeland. It felt like *Ma'apilim* at Camp Massad - the middle-of-the-night activity where we simulated the Jewish people coming into Israel in secret during the British mandate. That night always stirred in my young heart feelings of fear mixed with elation, and excitement at the prospect of reaching "Israel" — the bonfire after our trek through the dark woods. I remember hiding out in the forest with our group, trying to make the least noise as possible, so the "Brits" (counsellors) wouldn't find us. So that's how it felt being in a dark crowded bus with hostility outside but the warmth of my people inside. Looking around at my neighbours on the floor, returning their smiles, and having the soldier in the seat next to me shift slightly so I could lean on the seat, made me happy. Even in those moments of uncertainty, I felt an incredible sensation of shared experience, and it comforted me.

Tekoa itself is such a beautiful place. On Shabbat, I sat outside and read my book (The Alex Singer Story; about a young American who died defending Israel), overlooking Beit Lechem and the Arab villages around Tekoa. Periodically during the day, the voices of the *muezzin* from each of the four mosques within view would rise up to the sky, the notes of their individual prayers intertwining like Rapunzel's braids. Such beautiful melodies. I wish I didn't think of the dangers inherent in them. Barbara told me that sometimes those same beautiful voices are raised not in song and prayer but in supplication to kill the Jews... If only beauty could overcome the monster of hatred.

Later, on Shabbat, Ruthie and I took a walk around Tekoa, through the army base that is on the *Yishuv* and down to another area called Tekoa Bet (Tekoa #2). Tekoa Bet consists of a group of caravans situated overlooking a beautiful wadi that leads onwards through the desert to the Dead Sea. Behind the desert and sea, we could see the mountains of Jordan, and behind us lay the greener hills leading to Jerusalem. We sat on the rocks with our feet almost hanging over the wadi, and the shadows playing over the sand reminded me of the tragedy that took place there. Last year, two thirteen-year-old boys from Tekoa went for a hike through the wadi. A group of a dozen or more boys from one of the surrounding Arab villages attacked them; they dragged the two Jewish boys into a cave and stoned them to death. So again, I confronted the deception of beauty. When will beauty once again just be beauty? Why is it that humanity likes to dip its hands in blood and smear it over the landscape?

Although this email may sound sad and angry, it was intended to be the opposite. I had a truly exquisite time in Tekoa, and wish beyond words for peace so that one day I can raise children in a *Yishuv* like this one. Children and pets in Tekoa have such freedom, and they live amongst so many of their peers that life is good for them. I want such happiness for my children, and such health. The children of Tekoa look so healthy. Maybe it's the air!

All right, that's enough for now.

I miss you all, and will see you in one month!

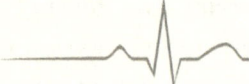

February 9, 2003

It's *Motzei Shabbat*, and time to write about what an adventure-filled Shabbat I had this week. Friday night I went to the Old City with Liz and Yoni, friends from Pardes. Liz is a fiery redhead who is one of the kindest people I've met here, and Yoni is Adee's roommate. We prayed *Kabbalat Shabbat* at the *Kotel* and then went for dinner at this guy Ezra's place after.

As we were sitting at the *Kotel*, on the stone bench beneath the row of Israeli flags, a beautiful white dove flew in out of nowhere. It was spectacular, as it flew around the *Kotel* plaza for a few minutes. The white dove flew past the *Kotel* with the golden Dome of the Rock behind it, then past the Israeli flag and all the Jews praying. She was then joined by a flock of pigeons, and another white dove. What an incredibly symbolic moment, or so it seemed; the perfect embodiment of hope for an elusive, yet fleeting, peace.

After prayers, we returned to the bench and waited for our friends. An orange-and-white cat came and sat on my lap. Stray cats in Israel are usually quite wary of people and won't come close, but this one curled up in my lap and fell asleep. We sat like that, keeping each other warm while I stroked her fur, for at least twenty minutes. It was a peaceful, sweet moment in time. It felt nice to give affection in such a simple way. I wished her *Shabbat Shalom*. Yoni said maybe she was a prophet reincarnated in a cat. One never knows who one will encounter in the Old City. The prophets of the bible all looked out at me from the cat's eyes. Then she wandered away and tried to curl up next to some other people sitting nearby, but they pushed her away, afraid of this sweet soul. Granted, she was a stray, smelly and dirty — but aren't we all that way sometimes? Don't we all search for someone to accept us, take care of us, despite our flaws? Wouldn't a prophet present itself in such a way — as a being we would rather ignore or shoo away than actually relate to? How many times might a messiah have tried to enter our reality, only to be chased away by our own fears? Perhaps the messiah wanders this earth, hidden, in perpetual torment as he/she tries so hard to reach us through boundaries of sensation and perception.

Last night I had a horrifyingly realistic dream. When I awoke I was surprised to find myself in my bed and not still in that plane of existence. We were on a *tiyul* with Pardes, to a *moshav* of some sort, in a forested area with single-floor condo-style residences to our right. We were walking toward the forest to go for a hike, when suddenly a woman appeared behind us. It was apparent she was a terrorist, and someone yelled, "Run!"

We ran toward the woods, but as I watched, she blew herself up in a bright white fire, releasing a cloud of gas that reached toward us. Before we could get away, another terrorist sprang out in front of us and blew up, again releasing a deadly cloud of gas. Gas surrounded us, and I could feel and taste it. It was tear gas, I suppose, because it felt just like the tear gas in Quebec City, at the protests I volunteered at as a medic in undergrad (Anti-Free Trade Area of the Americas protests in 2001). I felt it, even in the dream-space. I breathed it in, and it entered me and burned my insides. I stopped and looked around, and what I saw were two walls of gas on either side of me. Looking down those walls was like looking at train tracks that disappear into the distance, coming together. There was no way out, so I told everyone to run through one wall of gas toward the houses. We did, and reached one apartment that had an unlocked door. We all ran inside and closed the door behind us, but then a group of punk-looking boys began pounding on it. At first, I didn't want to let them in. I thought they looked scary and potentially dangerous. But then I realized we were in the middle of a war zone, a chemical attack, so I let them in. We shut the door again and prepared to hole up for a while. None of us had a gas mask (in this reality we still haven't received our masks...) and so the gas affected us. It was Shabbat, but I still used my phone to call my parents and tell them I was all right. Then the phone in the apartment rang, and it was the owners. They couldn't understand why there were people in their home, so I told them in Hebrew, "I am one of the people who are in your house in order to protect themselves." The family understood, and we settled in to wait for rescue.

The dream was so real. It felt like a horrible premonition. I guess that's what happens when you live in a place perpetually at war with its neighbours.

OK, I'm tired... going to bed.

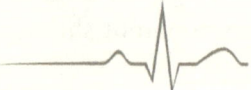

February 11, 2003, 12:44 a.m.

I am so confused. It's one of those times when I'm sad, and don't quite know why. Mid-cycle? Perhaps. Or perhaps it's that my life seems to be on a path I cannot quite control, or can control too much. I don't know what to do, where to be, who to be, or what to be. I'm in Israel, Yerushalayim, the place I had ached to be in for so long. My soul is here, but I'm starting to think my heart is somewhere else. I miss my family, but not only that, I miss Canada. I miss snow. I miss ice.

I miss blizzards and driving through whiteouts. I miss flying down a ski hill, singing inane songs in my head and waving to the tram at Jay Peak, imagining everyone is watching me racing. I miss slipping on the sidewalks, bundling up to walk outside, sitting in the kitchen with my feet on the heater and watching the snow outside. I miss feeling warm and drinking hot chocolate while seeing the chill outside. I miss it so much.

I am two people, two hearts, two wills. Jewish history tells of our exile from the land of Israel and our dispersion into the diaspora. What I am feeling — this is *Galut*, isn't it? The true punishment for whatever our people did two thousand years ago ... we were exiled physically, but we perpetuate that exile emotionally. Now that we have Israel for the Jewish people, perhaps the test becomes an individual one. Can we each rise to the challenge of breaking out of our "slave" mentality and leave our personal Egypts, as our ancestors did to escape Pharaoh? As beautiful and wonderful and comforting as Montreal may be, it is still my *Galut*. I must move forward if I am to be truly free, truly happy. I am chained to a land over the sea, and even though those chains may be warm and soothing rather than hard and choking, I must break them.

It's easy to say this. It's easy to start writing and let my subconscious take over, giving me truths even when I am not seeking for them. But it's a completely other thing to realize these truths in my deepest soul. It hurts! I want to be in two places at once. I want to be Sara who skis and skates and tumbles around in snow in Canada. But I also want to be Sara who lives so close to the *Kotel* that she can touch it every day...

What about my future? What will it bring? What is the destiny that is set out for me? What is the balance with my free will? Which path am I going to take? Persevere if I don't get into med school, and keep applying? Or recognize the possibility my path lies elsewhere? But maybe I am supposed to keep on the medicine path. How do I know?

Will I find love? How long must I feel so lonely? Is this part of my fate? Will I be alone? No, I feel I will meet my soulmate one day... I just wish I knew when.

I suppose it's all in God's hands, so I need to be patient. Keep going with my life and see what happens in the meantime.

I believe if I am a good person and do good things for humanity and for my people, good will come back to me.

Right?

I am going to *Shacharit* in the morning, so I'd better go to sleep. My friend Dyan's baby still hasn't come yet, and is on the small side. She's going to be induced Wednesday, so she asked me to pray for her. Tomorrow, I will do that. I wonder if there's a special prayer for such an instance?

Also, I have to remember to make an announcement tomorrow regarding the extremely high state of alert this week. The army caught three suicide bombers today, one with a twenty kg bomb ready to be detonated, entering into Jerusalem. The IDF has placed a compete shutdown on all the West Bank and Gaza until Friday, which means they are very anxious. So I'm going to tell everyone at Pardes tomorrow to be very careful this week.

Goodnight.

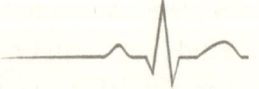

25

Best Decision of my Life

<u>February 17, 2003</u>

Shalom! Lots to write about today.

Last week on Wednesday, I went to work at MDA only to be sent home because there was no room on the ambulances. I put up a fuss, which is something I will never do again. I was in a horrible mood, having woken up at 5:45 a.m. after forcing myself to go to bed at 10 p.m., and now realizing my efforts were useless. Adee sent me a text message asking me to help him cook a yummy dinner that night, to which I immediately agreed. We cooked Asian-style lettuce wraps, stuffed with sautéed tofu cubes, celery, onions and carrots, with curried broccoli and cauliflower over rice. I was in heaven! We both just sat there admiring our work before eating it, and each bite was like biting into that perfect warm chocolate-chip cookie fresh out of an oven — in other words, delicious. It's at times like those I realize how lucky I am to have made such close friends here in Israel, and so quickly. Adee really took care of me by having me cook with him. He sensed that I was upset and helped me through it without having to talk about it.

Thinking back on the thoughts I had about not getting on an ambulance gives me mixed feelings. On the one hand, I am frustrated whenever the shifts are full, leaving no room for me. But then I realize that the shifts being full is a fantastic thing for the people of Israel, because it means that there are enough volunteers to staff MDA, with a surplus! So it is not fair of me to react with anger to a situation that is beneficial to my country and my people. Having to go home because there is no room for me is a good thing, and I need to adjust my attitude and emotional response to take that into account. Phew! Self-psychoanalysis is a heavy and sticky thing to do.

This past Shabbat, we went on another Pardes trip, this time to Zippori and Mitzpeh Hoshaya, in the Lower Galil. Zippori is a National Park, and is basically one huge archaeological dig spanning at least two thousand years of history. We visited the synagogue and stood gazing at its mosaic, with the images of our Temple and ancient way of life. It was beautiful. From the glass window of the building we stood in, we could see the modern synagogue of Hoshaya across the valley. Two thousand years of Jewish history spanned that gulf of olive trees. The fascinating thing about Zippori is the intensity of its pagan roots. Many of the mosaics we saw were most definitely not monotheistic. It's interesting to contemplate the relationship Jews and pagans had in Mishnaic times. Mishnaic... let me explain that word. Judaism has its basis in many books, such as the Tanach (*Torah* - Five Books of Moses, Neviim - Prophets, Ketuvim - Writings), Mishnah, Gemarah, etc. The Mishnah is the codification of Jewish oral law and tradition as compiled by Rabbi Yehudah HaNassi, who lived in Zippori hundreds of years ago. The *Mishnah* itself was compiled in Zippori. Given that I am spending this year studying the Mishnah (amongst so many other subjects), walking the very stone streets that Rabbi Yehudah HaNassi stepped on is a very special experience. The mosaics and remnants of Mishnah-era life in Zippori gave me a taste (in the short time we were there) of what Jewish existence must have been like, and what led to the compilation of the Mishnah. I truly believe that in order to understand our books of law well, we must delve into the lives and times of the men who collected them and put them together in a bound, readable state of being. I wish I had more time in Zippori to get to know my ancestors.

Mitzpeh Hoshaya... what a beautiful place. We stayed with host families for Shabbat, and it was a thrilling experience. Shoshana and I stayed with the Eldar family, who have five children (three of whom were home this weekend: ten-year-old Amir, eight-year-old Yuval and four-year-old Adee). Ne'amah and Eyal (the parents) made us feel so welcomed. They spoke no English, so we spent the full Shabbat speaking only Hebrew. On Saturday, the Pardes students went on a walk through the fields between Zippori and Hoshaya - it was spectacular. Wildflowers dominated the landscape with reds, purples, whites, yellows, pinks... The *Kalaniyot* (a type of flower that is protected in Israel) were astounding. It was a very relaxing, perfect way to spend my Shabbat.

On our way to Zippori, we first stopped at a place that will be for eternity one of pilgrimage: the grave of Ilan Ramon, Israel's first astronaut. Two weeks ago, on February 1, 2003, Ilan's life and growth were tragically cut down when the space shuttle Columbia exploded minutes from the moment he would have embraced his family. Ilan's grave, covered in wreaths and flowers, gifts and stones, lies peacefully on a ridge of the cemetery in Nahalal, where men and women such as Moshe Dayan and other great Israeli heroes are buried. Together they form some sort of mystical shield over Israel, or so I hope. The gravesite itself is a beautiful testimonial to an Israeli hero, in a *Keren Kayemet Le'Israel* (Jewish National Fund) forest on a hill overlooking the Galilee.

We said *Tehillim* for Ilan and read a poem in his honour. We let the driving, icy rain take our tears with it as it watered his grave, and each standing there huddled in his or her own thoughts to keep warm. When Adee read a Psalm called *Mimaamakim* (from the depths), an Israeli man, also standing by the grave, joined in to help him. The intensity of Israel is revealed at these moments, when complete strangers connect through the ancient words of our people and the depth of sorrow.

Ilan's gravesite was covered in so many flowers the tombstone beneath was not visible. I added a pinecone and a stone to the pile of wishes. What a man – truly a hero, and one that we do not have the honour of receiving in this world very often.

Thursday night we had a *hishtalmut* session at MDA, for the war. It was four hours of Hebrew; technical, scientific Hebrew. I shocked myself by understanding almost everything, laughing at the jokes, and by taking eight pages of notes in Hebrew! It was fascinating to learn the Hebrew terms for neurotransmission and chemical warfare agents. The *hishtalmut* covered what MDA and other public services will do in the event of a war, and we learned what our roles would be should that day come. We filled out sheets with our details: name, address, phone number, location should war break out, willingness to volunteer at that time, marital status, etc. They taught us all the protocols for a state of emergency in Israel, how to react to and treat victims of a chemical or biological attack, and how to protect ourselves. Someone tried on the big green suit, to show us what we need to wear in the ambulances, complete with a space-age gas mask.

Later, Yael informed me that foreign volunteers will not be allowed on the ambulances during a war, but we will be called upon to help in the stations and at the public shelters. We will be giving first aid at the shelters, handing out antibiotics if needed, etc. I'm not 100 per cent sure what our job will entail, but I am ready to help in whatever way possible.

Last night Shoshana and I took care of a cat that was hit by a car. One front leg was broken, and I think she had either a head injury (internal) or a spinal injury. When she got herself standing, she ran around in a small circle, confused and unable to straighten out. We called the city to come and pick her up, to either be taken to a vet or to be put down. I would have loved to have kept her, but she was a street cat, unvaccinated, wild. I don't know what my housemates would have said. Enough with the excuses! I should have kept her. It eats me away inside that I let them take her and put her down, but she was deteriorating and in severe shock. I sat with her on the cold ground for an hour while Shoshana tried to feed her some milk, and I covered her in a towel so she wouldn't freeze. It was highly emotional. I was petting her head (with gloves on) to let her know someone cared, and to relieve her anxiety. I didn't know she actually was responding until the man came to take her away. When she saw him coming she stood up, hid behind me and then put her head in my lap. She was asking me for help, and I picked her up, put her in a cage and said goodbye. What did I do? Was it wrong? Did I sentence her to death without giving her a chance to heal? I know if this situation ever comes up again, that cat is coming home with me, no matter the consequences. I just hope this cat is in a better place than the cold, wild, and dirty Jerusalem streets.

Being with the cat taught me more about Israeli society. As we sat there with the cat, on the ground outside the Ministry of Health, looking like a couple of bums, a group of middle-aged men and women came over to talk to us. They felt for the cat, calling her *miskenah*, and asking what had happened to her. Then a big, gruff-looking man came over and told us he was going to bring us cups for the milk — and he did. We then continued feeding her with ease. An Arab man pulled up in his truck and told us the cat had been there since morning, and that he was embarrassed at not having helped her (since he has three dogs at home and was scared she might be contagiously ill). He told us "*Kol Hakavod.*" I continue to be struck by how in a country so ravaged by pain, there is so much affection and caring just waiting to be brought to the surface.

Today at MDA was wild. I'll just tell you about the last call. We were called to take an Arab girl from a hospital in Jerusalem back to her house in Hevron so she could recuperate from surgery. First, we went back to the station and switched into a bulletproof ambulance (used whenever one is going to cross the green line or go into a particularly dangerous place), and then we picked her and her mother up. We then drove out of Jerusalem, on the Tunnel Road, past Efrat and through Gush Etzion, until we reached the *machsom* outside Hevron. We dropped them off at that point, and did not go any further; they took a bus the rest of the way. Even at MDA, there is a limit as to how far into the Shtachim we will go; there is a line after which one has truly taken their lives into their own hands. I felt pretty well protected inside the ambulance *memugan*, especially with the soldiers and the checkpoints we went through. However, I did feel bad that we couldn't accompany this family all the way back to their home, as they deserved.

I truly feel that these kinds of experiences are necessary in my growth as a person, as a caregiver, as a doctor-to-be and as a Jew. I am curious about our cousins. I want to see how they live and how they function, and I want to be privileged enough to see again such beautiful marble eyes as I saw in the girl's mother today. Her whole soul shone through her eyes and smiled at me. Thousands of years of strife were forgotten in the connection between our *neshamot*. I want to see more of that. I want to feel that indescribable sensation of being emotionally punched in the stomach so that you lose your breath and realize the gulf you thought was so wide is really just a narrow wadi that can be crossed through the heart. I'm not really sure what I meant to say, but sometimes my heart speaks through my keyboard and I don't quite control what comes out.

Please accept this attempt to describe to you the beauty and complexity of this incredible country and its people. Coming here was the best decision of my life.

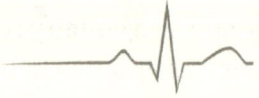

26

Snowstorm

February 21, 2003

Shalom everyone,

It's my second to last Shabbat here before I go back to Montreal for a month. As much as I am excited to go home and see everyone, especially my family (I MISS YOU), I am very sad to have to leave Israel. Especially in time of crisis for the country. But I do feel like I've helped Israel and her people somewhat in the time that I've been here. There is so much more I want to do, but life is life. I will be back on April 2.

Yesterday, along with five other foreign volunteers at MDA, I drove to the main MDA warehouse near Tel Aviv and helped with war preparation. We assembled gas masks for the ambulance drivers and medics, and put together other war-time supplies. I can't tell you many details, because as my friends reminded me yesterday, revealing information about things such as supplies may compromise Israel's security situation. One never knows, right? Better safe than sorry.

What I will tell you is this: preparing and assembling gas masks for ambulance crews gave me an intense feeling of satisfaction. Finally, I feel like I truly helped Israel. As I put batteries in and checked each mask, I sensed I was holding a life in my hands, and the lives of many others in a growing circle around me. If a gas mask functions properly, a medic can leave the ambulance in a chemical or biological weapons attack, and go out to save lives. If the mask fails to work, the medic will be stuck in the ambulance, and might even die. Standing in the warehouse with other foreign volunteers, assembling lifesaving materials, I felt my connection and relevance to Israel and the Jewish people intensifying until my heart felt so full it could burst. Days like yesterday make me remember that life is so beautiful — even in times of war and anxiety, a small act of helping can make a person happier than at any other time in their life. I can't explain the feeling.

Shabbat Shalom U'Mevorach (whether you celebrate it Friday, Saturday, Sunday, or not at all).

I miss you.

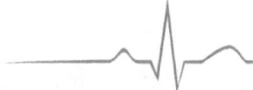

February 26, 2003

Shalom everyone!

The past two days I've had off from both Pardes and MDA, because Jerusalem is under attack — from snow! We have received so much snow that there are inches still on the ground. I was at MDA on Monday when the first flakes and hailstones began to fall, and rapidly built up into a full-blown snowstorm worthy of Montreal. The wind was intense, whipping the snow into walls of blinding flakes. Snow fell throughout the night on Monday, so that at 5:15 a.m. a friend of mine sent me a text saying "No school!" I got up and looked out the window to see the white world that I've been missing this winter. I took a picture and snuggled back up under my covers for a well-earned sleep-in. At 9, my friend Avi called to ask me to come make pancakes with him and Shaiel, but I declined in favour of sleep. At 11:15 my friend Elana called, followed again by Shaiel, telling me to get up and come meet them in Gan HaPaamon (the Bell Gardens) to play in the snow. So Liz and I walked down Derech Beit Lechem in the snow and sleet, getting our feet soaked in the process. About thirty minutes later, we were in the middle of a great snow fight, rolling around on the ground and having a fantastic time.

After playing for a while like children, the six of us trekked down to the Old City to take pictures of it in the snow. It was beautiful — what a sight, to see the walls of Jerusalem and the *Kotel* white with snow. It's the kind of sight that some people never see in their lifetimes. What a privilege.

It's funny how in Israel, the tiniest bit of snow shuts down the entire country. The public transportation wasn't running, everything was closed, and taxis were scarce. Jerusalem was a ghost town.

But it's on days like yesterday that one can do things here that we would never do on a regular busy day - like walk around the Muslim quarter of the Old City and visit the Church of the Holy Sepulchre. Adee, Elana, and I did just that. We took pictures of kids making snowmen and snow forts in the middle of ancient paths, and we walked alleyways I haven't set foot in since the start of the *matzav*. It was a scary but exciting hour we spent trudging along, and I am so happy we did it.

Finally, we arrived at the *Kotel* — Adee took us to an observation point above Aish Hatorah, a religious institution, facing the Wall. We took some incredible photos and then walked down to the snow-covered plaza. By that time we were freezing and wet, so we hopped in a cab back to Adee's.

We bought wine, hot chocolate, bread and cheese, and Adee had made split-pea soup. We exchanged our wet clothes for Adee and Yoni's dry stuff, put our boots and shoes in front of the heaters to dry (steaming!), and curled up on the couches. Our whole *Chevrah* ended up there, eating, drinking, and relaxing for hours.

Finally, at around 10:30, we got a call from someone at Pardes, telling us we were needed to come help bail out the flooded rooms. We all shlepped over with buckets to find two classrooms full of an inch or two of water. The ceiling had a gigantic crack and the snow above was melting into the building. We spent hours bailing out the place and made shifts to come back throughout the night to empty buckets. It's amazing how a community pulls together in times of crisis, and it's at times like those that you realize who truly is dependable and who is not. We had some people refuse to come and help - and then those of us who chose to come back for a few shifts and clean up. What a night. Today my housemates and I spent the day playing cards and relaxing, while outside the snow sat white and soft and so beautiful.

Jerusalem on a snow day is beyond description.

I miss you all, but now I've got my fill of snow.

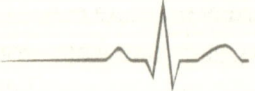

27

Interlude - Home

<u>March 5, 2003, 9:30 a.m. Canadian time</u>

Somewhere over Ontario

Here I am, flying back to Montreal for a month of medical school interviews and family time. I didn't want to leave Israel, but this trip is necessary not only for my future but for my own emotional satisfaction and happiness at seeing Mom, Dad and my sisters.

It feels remarkably different, almost foreign, to be back in this society. I have adjusted so well to the Israeli mode of being, that it seems like that is my natural way. In Israel, people may be rude and pushy sometimes, but you know that underneath the tough *Sabra* exterior lies such caring for each other that sometimes feeling that energy makes my heart almost burst. Here in Canada, I do not feel that depth of emotion, that heart-charge, between people. Everyone seems to live their lives as separate individuals on unique paths to unique destinies. Sometimes I view the Jewish People, and even more so those of us already in Israel, as a group who are moving toward a communal fate. *Am Yisrael* has survived so many seemingly insurmountable obstacles. We continue to fly to some unknown but much-imagined destiny that we believe exists, and because we are cognizant of our peoplehood and unity, we care that much more for the outcomes of each other's lives.

To illustrate, let me tell a classic, only in Israel story:

Yesterday I was riding the bus back from my trek to the Kotel (I went to say goodbye and put a note in for a friend). There was a guy sitting in front of me who was giggling to himself, for no apparent reason; no reading material, no headphones, no cell phone. He was hysterical, laughing to himself, cracking himself up, and other people on the bus were starting to notice. Two girls sitting further up the bus started giggling as well. Soon it was uncontrollable, and the girl beside me and I were both laughing too. Within moments, everyone on the bus was giggling to themselves! As the original laughing girls were getting off the bus, one of them turned to the guy and asked him politely what was so funny, because everyone wanted to be let in on the joke. He couldn't answer, just laughed and laughed; it must have been some private thought. So the girl thanked him for giving us all something to be happy about, and walked off the bus. It was a wonderful experience, to have everyone in a scary situation (riding the bus in Israel) just start laughing for no reason and with open hearts. I felt invigorated, inspired, and more alive than ever as I stepped off the bus with a wave back at the boy who had made us all smile for just a moment in our hectic lives. I thank him with all my heart for those minutes.

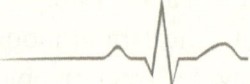

March 20, 2003 12:15 a.m.

Sitting on the bed in our friends the Sinclair's house in Vermont, about to go to bed.

We (Mom, Annie and I) came here two days ago to ski and "take a break from the world" as Mom puts it. No such luck, as the US began attacking Iraq a few hours ago. It's Gulf War #2, only this time I'm not a sixth grader writing letters to Israeli kids, but a skilled medic heading to Israel to help, on April 2. My family obviously doesn't want me to go, but I feel the obligation and the instinctual need to be there. Perhaps Israel will not be affected at all by this war, although I find it hard to believe. We'll see.

I'm conflicted over my feelings toward this invasion. On the one hand, I know Saddam Hussein's regime must be taken out (like the Taliban were in Afghanistan). Hussein possesses weapons of mass destruction capable of destroying the world as we know it. And he's crazy enough to use them. So we must get him before he gets us.

But so many people will likely die. So many innocents. And so many more will lose all they have, and be forced to flee a bombarded, burning land. The desert will be deserted, and so much more barren.

What is morally right?

What is just?

What will provide a firmer and lasting calm?

Will we find peace?

Will we suffer the terrorist reprisals in *our* cities?

What about Israel?

Are we worrying for nothing?

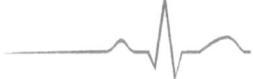

April 1, 2003

Dear Everyone,

Tomorrow I am flying back to Israel. I'm very excited but at the same time I know how much I will miss my family. I'm sitting here at our computer, trying not to cry or let the conflicting emotions overwhelm me.

When I return to Jerusalem, I will write.

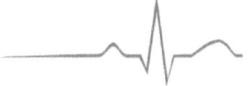

28

A Dream Fulfilled

<u>April 2, 2003</u>

GREAT NEWS!

I woke up to a phone call today from Ben Gurion University - I got into the International Medicine program that is run in conjunction with Columbia University!

I AM GOING TO BE A DOCTOR!!!!!!!!!!

Thanks to every one of you who supported me and helped me through this long admissions process.

You're all so close to my heart.

Still waiting on McGill...

Miss you all.

Love

Sara

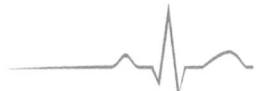

29

Chamsin

<u>April 4, 2003</u>

Shabbat Shalom!

Here I am back in my cozy apartment in Jerusalem, but what a different Jerusalem it is. A month makes a tremendous difference here. When I left, there was still some snow littering the streets, and it was cold. Last night was tropical, and today is stifling. Tomorrow will be even worse, apparently. We're in the middle of what's called a *Chamsin*, which sounds like it comes from the Hebrew word for hot (*cham*). The *Chamsin* is a weather phenomenon; a hot, dry, dusty, desert wind. The forecasters predicted a dust storm tomorrow in Jerusalem, so I will be super careful with my asthma.

Other than the weather and the fact that Shabbat is super late to start, things are about the same. I'm having dinner and lunch for Shabbat with friends, and we're going on a *tiyul* to the Golan Heights from Sunday to Tuesday. I'm very excited to see everyone again - apparently they've all missed me, which makes me feel great.

Regarding the war situation, surprisingly, things are pretty calm here. No one is carrying their gas masks around, and the guard at the supermarket laughed when he checked my knapsack and saw I was carrying mine. But I am going to keep it with me all the time, because I promised my family that I'd be super safe, and I also want to protect myself just in case the improbable happens. Don't worry about me; I think Israel will come out of this newest war untouched.

I miss you all!

Oh, by the way - my mom is coming to Israel in May. Isn't that fantastic? I'm super proud of her; she's coming on a trip for foreign doctors who can come to Israel in times of crisis. MDA will train them in how the Israeli medical system functions. Luckily, Mom will spend her first Shabbat here with me.

Mom, I am so proud of you and can't wait till you get here!

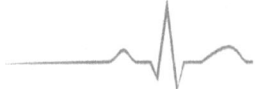

April 11, 2003 12:45 a.m.

Shalom everyone!

It's been a week since I returned to this incredibly breathtakingly beautiful country, and I can't believe I was gone for a month. It feels as if I never left.

Last Friday, my friend Laurie invited me to a nice small Shabbat dinner at her house; just six of us around a cozy table. It was just what I needed. Being welcomed back so warmly by my friends here has been an exceptional experience; it reminds me how quickly people bond together as friends or even family. I feel so honoured and blessed to have people here who love me and watch out for me.

In the early morning on Sunday, we at Pardes left on a *tiyul* to the Golan Heights up at the Northern extreme of Israel. Stunning scenery greeted us as we drove first through the Jordan Valley and then up past the Kinneret and Beit Shean. The bus then climbed a twisting, steep, dizzyingly high road up into the mountains of the Golan, after which the land opened up into a huge long plateau of green fields and orchards. The Golan Heights is essentially one long strip of raised farmland and hiking spots, but the sad part about it is that when the Golan was under Syrian control, they mined it heavily. Although they both possess the same natural features, far from being the safe space Switzerland is, the Golan is one big minefield. The Israeli forces managed to de-mine many areas that are now inhabited and used agriculturally, and they also cleared some of the most fantastic hiking spots in the country.

Let me back up for those of you who are not familiar with the Golan Heights and the history of this place. Jews have lived in the Golan since before our ancestors built the First Temple; literally thousands of years. In recent history, however, the Golan was under Syrian control until June 1967. From the heights the Syrian soldiers would terrorize Jewish settlements beneath them, in Israel. Shelling was continuous and life below the Golan was exceedingly dangerous. So in 1967, the Israeli army annexed the Golan for many reasons, primarily because of the strategic nature of the place and to ensure secure defensible borders for Israel.

Moving on from history and politics.... We spent three days hiking in one of the most beautiful places I've ever been privileged enough to see. Trekking through long river valleys, standing in awe before tumbling waterfalls over basalt or limestone rocks, swimming in freezing cold Mount Hermon water in a pool surrounded by flowers... these moments will remain etched in my memory forever.

For those of you familiar with Israeli hikes, we did Nachal El-Al, Nachal Zavitan, Nachal Iyyon (by Metulla) and more. We drove through the Hula Valley, past the base of Mount Hermon (Israel's ski hill, believe it or not, still covered partially in snow), below Har Dov (Israeli military base on a mountaintop overlooking Syria), through Kiryat Shemona (a small village often shelled by Hezbollah, terrorist group in Lebanon) and by Metulla. Where once I visited the Good Fence, a sometime border crossing between Lebanon and Israel, there was virtually nothing but a stark cold-looking fence. In the past there were always tourists, and soldiers on both sides of the fence ready to pose for pictures. Not so anymore. In Nachal Iyyon, we saw enormous amounts of water cascading in four huge waterfalls, reminding us of what a bountiful winter Israel had this year.

On our last day, we went kayaking (really just inflatable rafts for two people) down the Jordan River right before it pours into the Kinneret. It was fantastic! Of course none of us had any idea what we were doing, but we splashed each other and had a really fun time. After kayaking we prayed *Minchah* and in the middle I saw two army helicopters fly over the ridge nearby. I waved at them (I know, I'm a child) and an instant later they each released something that flashed and then was lost in a cloud of smoke. I have no idea what that was, but I assume they must have been practicing manoeuvres (unless, of course, they were waving back at me in their way).

Wednesday morning I went to Beit Hanassi (the President's House) here in Jerusalem. As a foreign volunteer for MDA, I was invited along with four others to a ceremony for "lone soldiers", *Hayalim Bodedim*, who are here in Israel without their families. Many of these soldiers hadn't seen their parents in years, given that the soldiers had made Aliyah and their parents couldn't afford to. Most of these soldiers were from the Former Soviet Union and South America. At the ceremony, they were reunited with family; the Jewish Agency paid for the families to come visit for a short period. It was a very emotional, moving day. I met Sallai Meridor, president of the Jewish Agency, and President Moshe Katsav and his wife. There were photo ops, so when I get copies I'll send them on.

Phew. Other than all that excitement, life is relatively normal and quiet here. We have three weeks off from Pardes for Passover break, and I'm going to Tekoa to be with friends for Passover. I'm leaving here Tuesday morning and will probably come back on Sunday. I'm very excited to have a Seder here in Israel. Passover is the holiday of freedom for the Jewish People, and really a holiday about aliyah. Passover is the story of our exodus from slavery in Egypt, our journey through the desert to Mount Sinai and then our arrival in Israel. What a special thing, to celebrate a holiday about Jewish freedom in the place where I feel the most Jewish and the most free! What a gift, to eat the Pesach feast here in the land that we were promised and given. I know how lucky I am, and I appreciate every second of this present time.

One more quick tidbit before I let you go: I have a new roommate. The other night I noticed some twigs in my enclosed balcony and realized that a bird was building a nest in my bookshelf! I rapidly removed my important possessions from the bookshelf and put down some comfy tissue paper and padding for the nest to sit on. I picked up the half-built nest and moved it to its new location. This morning I was woken up by loud cooing and wings flapping nearby; looking out the window into the porch, I saw one dove sitting on the fully built nest, and its mate perched in the window. As I go to bed tonight, I will look over at the resting bird sitting on her nest, and know that she, too, is living her brief life to the fullest. In a few days I suppose there will be the two eggs of her clutch laid in the nest, and within a month her babies will fledge and fly away.

What a wonderful world I live in; even with all the suffering around us, I still feel happy and alive.

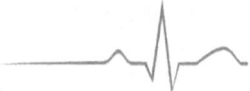

April 16, 2003

Got to Tekoa this morning and I've been helping Barbara cook for Pesach. I went over to the base to see my friend Nadav, who's stationed here for a few months. Nadav is the son of my Rabbi, Ron, and his wife Carmela, who was my grade school teacher. He is a few years younger than I am, and moved to Israel to join the army. He used to be this adorable little round kid, and now he's tall, dark and handsome. Visiting him at the army base was really strange, intense, fascinating, but frightening. We sat in his room (he lives with three other guys in the infirmary) for an hour and a half, talking. Then he was called to go out on a mission, so he took me to see his jeep. He showed me all the equipment, including his huge, heavy flak vest, his radio (he's the radio guy), his night vision goggles, etc. The whole time, of course, he was carrying his gun - a huge M-16 with a grenade launcher attached.

It felt really scary to be around all that weaponry, but more scary knowing Nadav has to use it. He gets shot at, people try to kill him, all the time. That's what being a soldier in the Israel Defense Forces is like these days.

As Nadav and I were standing around, we watched the other soldiers inspecting a car that was just stoned on the way up to Tekoa. The young couple and their baby were fine; I talked for a minute with the mom. Their windshield was a mess, cracked and cratered.

They're lucky to be alive.

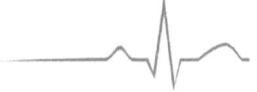

30

May All Your Dreams Come True

April 17, 2003

I GOT ACCEPTED TO MCGILL!!!!!!!!!!

Love,

Sara

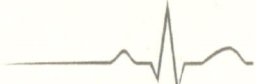

Friday April 18, 2003

Shabbat Shalom and Chag Sameach!

It's Friday afternoon before Shabbat Pesach and I want to send out an ecstatic email. As you all know, a couple of nights ago, I found out that I was accepted to McGill's medical school. What many of you may not know is that I've been working towards this my whole life. Since I was a child, I knew I wanted to be a doctor, and I decided I wanted to follow in my parents' footsteps at McGill. My parents met there and fell in love, and as one of my smart aunties reminded me - without McGill, I wouldn't be here. It's been a long road to this day and I feel like all of my hard work paid off. I feel blessed - I know that without someone upstairs looking out for me, I might not be in this place right now. It's an amazing feeling to recognize that life can work out, and to know that what we strive for and dream about can become a reality.

Let me tell you the incredible story of how I found out...

It was Wednesday, April 16, and the acceptances were due to be posted online. Passover was quickly approaching, and no news. So my mother called the admissions office, and they told her that if she called back at 2 p.m., they would tell her my status. But 2 p.m. Montreal time is 9 p.m. Israel time, past the point when I could answer the phone and pushing into the Seder hours. So my mother and I decided on a code: one ring on my phone meant I was on the waiting list, two rings signalled acceptance, and no rings indicated refusal.

At 9:05, my phone rang once. I waited, and told those around me at the Seder table that being waitlisted would be fantastic (I truly wasn't expecting more!). Then my phone rang again! I jumped up from the table, screaming, and started crying. Everyone was so excited (there were seventeen of us at the table) and hugging me. It was the best way to find out, short of being with my family at that moment.

So I will attend McGill in August, and begin the long, hard journey towards the day when I can call myself a doctor. I don't know how long that will take — the four years of learning is probably not enough — but it feels incredible to be on the path.

There is so much more to write. Thank you so much to all of you who stood by me and believed in me (even when I really didn't!). Thank you to those of you who wrote my letters of reference and rooted for me at McGill. Thank you to everyone who cares about me.

Shabbat is starting soon — I'll send out another email on Sunday about my time over Passover, in Tekoa. For now, let me say this: Passover is the Jewish holiday of liberation, of starting a life-altering and destiny-changing journey into an untracked desert towards our Torah and our future in Israel. God made us a promise to take us out of heartbreak and into happiness, and He pulled through for us in every way. This Pesach is extra special for me, both being here in Jerusalem and also having crossed my own Red Sea into my own desert. I feel like I am about to tread through burning hot sand under a scorching sun, with scorpions and wild beasts. It's certain that I will lose faith sometimes, but so did our people at the very mountain where we received the core of our beliefs. I know that I, like my ancestors before me, will continue on my journey and make my own way to my own promised land — both figuratively and literally. I will become who I know I am meant to be, and I will also come back here to the place I love.

I wish the same for all of you. May all your dreams come true.

Miss you all.

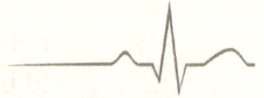

31

Pesach in Tekoa, a Lone Soldier, and Murder

Saturday night, April 19, 2003

Time to write about my Pesach in Tekoa...

On Tuesday, I took the bulletproof bus up to Tekoa, a settlement in the West Bank that I've written to you all about before. I went to spend Pesach with my friends in their beautiful house, with a bunch of other Montrealers that I haven't seen in a long time. We cooked and cooked and cooked and then cleaned and cleaned and cleaned till we were all exhausted. It was so much fun to be in such an active and happy place. The Seder was joyful, long enough (till about 2 a.m. I think) and with tons of yummy food. It was remarkable to be in Israel on such a holiday, the holiday of our liberation and entrance into the Promised Land. To sing "Next Year in Jerusalem" and the Israeli anthem while looking out the windows into the very land my voice was praising and yearning for - that's a feeling unlike any other. My heart soared while singing about longing for Jerusalem while being only fifteen minutes away from the heartbeat of that city.

On the first day of Passover, Thursday, we lay out on the grass tanning and reading books. It was really relaxing. Wednesday before the Seder, Aviva and I took a bunch of food up to the soldiers at the base in Tekoa. My friend Nadav is there now, and it was great to visit with him. Aviva had to go, so I sat around with Nadav and a bunch of soldiers while they gorged themselves on proper food for once. A very satisfying feeling, and extremely special, to bring Passover food to the very men who are protecting my country and keeping us free. These boys hadn't had such good food in a really long time! You should have seen it — five boys in their khakis sitting around a table in the infirmary (an old caravan) chowing down on cold chicken, potato balls and salad. It really felt good to be there with them.

I don't know how to explain the emotions inside stirred up by my repeated visits to the base. Fear, pride, joy, agony, so much and in such a complex mix. Hard to know what to do with those feelings.

Take, for instance, when Nadav had me walk him to his jeep, as the soldiers were being called out to a mission. He showed me his equipment, he put on his equipment, and showed off the various "toys" at his disposal. Shivers ran up and down my spine as he took me on this little tour. As proud as I am of him, as important as these soldiers are to me, I was so scared. I didn't want him to go. I didn't want these young kids, just a few years younger than me, to risk their beautiful bodies and souls on such dangerous pursuits. But at the same moment, I wished them a safe and successful mission, and hoped that they would continue to protect me and my people.

Living in this rolling, changing, turbulent country is like throwing one's emotions into the washing machine with a pair of old dirty sneakers covered in mud. You know that you're going to be soiled, hurt, turned over and over and drowned in pain, but you also know that through it all, you are getting cleansed and washed and ready for whatever the next day has to bring. My heart and soul feel like they are being renewed every moment that I am here, and for that, I am so grateful. I feel so lucky and blessed to have someone like Nadav in my life, to call him a friend, because to me what he does is true heroism. Through three years of hell, he has managed to keep his principles, to stand by his values and, above all, to stay human. He has grown intellectually and spiritually, out of his little boy's life and into a real man who knows what matters in life. Carmela and Rabbi Ron — you should really be so proud. I am.

Phew. Well, that turned into a different email than I expected, but nevertheless a very important message to you all. We have an army here that respects the enemy, and treats them as human beings. In my own words, I told you a story of one soldier, here alone without his family to help him, thrust into a war zone of unimaginable moral complexity. I want you to understand this small glimpse of him, and I want you to care about him. If I accomplished that at all, I am glad.

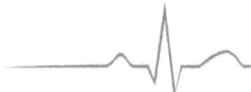

April 20, 2003 1:37 a.m.

I don't think I ever wrote about walking in the wadi of Tekoa, and those moments are vital to share.

Ruthie took a bunch of us for a walk to the wadi just outside Tekoa, a dry riverbed winding through the desert hills like a canyon. Kobi Mandel and Yosef Ishran, two thirteen-year-old Tekoa boys, were brutally murdered in this very spot early in this *intifada*. They went for a hike just as we were doing, two best friends out to have a peaceful, quiet day. That was never to be, as about thirteen young adults and teenagers from the neighbouring Arab villages ambushed them. They were dragged into a cave and stoned to death with rocks in the fists of boys barely older than they were. A savage and sick killing of innocents.

So on Pesach, holiday of freedom and exodus from suffering, a group of us (six or so) walked to the wadi. Many people from Tekoa go there to hike and relax, so we felt safe enough. Most people who go to the wadi bring *neshek* for protection, but we didn't have any with us. On the way down, soldiers passing us in a jeep told us to be careful. In fact, we didn't go all the way down into the wadi, because one of our number was afraid of the steep slopes. We sat on the hillside and split into two smaller groups; one to stay with the girl who was afraid, and one to make a short foray onwards. We traded afterwards, so that each of us would get a chance to see more of the spectacularly beautiful scenery.

Directly across from us, we could see the cave where the boys met their tragic fates. It was surreal to sit in such an overwhelmingly splendid spot, so tranquil, and know what happened there. With the same breath, I tasted fresh grass, wildflowers, and blood. With the same sweep of my eyes I saw people hiking, bees buzzing in tall stands of blossoms, the mountains of Jordan, the settlements of Nokdim and Tekoa, and a cave dark with a spectre of winking Death at the entrance. Closing my eyes I heard the thrilling calls of birds all around, blending with the buzz of the busy bees, songs being hummed under my friends' breaths, and the distant thunder of airplanes - all mixed in one twisted jam session with screaming and crying and the dull thud of rock against flesh. Why do we have such tragedy and brutality in our world? What is the reasoning behind such torment? And how is it that such evil can be juxtaposed, indeed framed, by the background of such an incredibly beautiful place? The land I walk on here is holy to so many; Israel is a place of spiritual elevation, unlike any other in the universe. How can we be so high and yet so low all at once? Will there ever be a balance, and if so, what will we have to sacrifice to achieve it? Isn't the blood of our children so much more than enough? Isn't *Hashem* the same God who told us He does not wish for human sacrifice? Then why is the tribute still so high?

Tekoa is a wild place of stark contrasts; it has captured my heart inconceivably. How do I feel so refreshed in a place that is so hotly disputed? Why do I feel so thrillingly free and happy when I walk the streets of this place, when deep down I know I am in danger each moment of my time there?

Who knows? I have no clue how the inner workings of my heart, soul, or mind function. Next year I will learn the physical logistics, but I would need a private audience with *Hashem* to get the rest of my questions answered. I think that would take a while.

For now, all I can do is follow the path my heart takes me on, and hope my instincts are correct. But what do you do with the cave? Do you walk up to it, face the evil within, and fight it with all your might? Do you turn away and pretend the cave is not there? I feel that for me, the best course of action is this: I must see the cave, approach it, witness the terror within, acknowledge its existence and store that inside my soul. I don't know yet how to fight it, but I must recognize it and maybe one day I will have the tools to understand it and break down its powers. One day. But not yet.

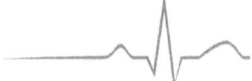

April 22, 2003   7:22 p.m.

I'm sitting on a lounge chair at one end of the Tel Aviv beach, by the Dolphinarium discotheque, where a suicide bombing took place last year.

The sun is setting, and the sky is red fire above raging green surf. There are surfers on the water, a kid playing in the sand next to me, friends to be with and music to groove to. The sound of the Mediterranean is complemented by the beat behind me. I am surrounded by sensory gifts. Planes are flying above me, small and large, just missing each other.

It is astonishing to feel such peace and rest in a place where such fiery hell rained down a year ago. I hope the beauty and silence of the sea breeze can comfort the souls of our kids killed here not long ago.

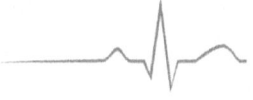

32

Choose Your Own Adventure

April 25, 2003

Med school decision time

Shabbat Shalom,

So I'm sitting here by the phone, with my Ben Gurion paperwork on my lap, trying to muster the ability to call and turn down my acceptance. I paid the tuition deposit for McGill this morning, feeling euphoric that all my dreams have come true. But I can't shake this nagging feeling that it's not quite right. Must be because I'm leaving Israel again, after being so happy here and finding such beauty amid madness. This is cyclical in my life; I come here, feeling like I can never leave, only to get back on a plane and fly out of the place I love the most. How do you choose paths in life? I feel like I'm in a "Choose Your Own Adventure" storybook from my childhood, where at the end of each page you pick between two options of where the story will lead. Each option has a different denouement and a different ending; sometimes it is relatively easy to know which path is the best, but often it's a struggle between desires and conscience. This is how I feel right now. The most rational thing to do would be go to McGill. I've even rationalized leaving Israel by saying that I won't be in debt at the end and can come back here sooner. I know ultimately McGill is the right choice financially and stability-wise, and I've wanted this my whole life. But I just can't shake the feeling that this is not quite right. I know I said that already... but bear with me on my ramblings. I have to work this out for myself.

I know I can come back here during breaks and in the summer, especially considering all the money I'll save by going to McGill, so Israel is not lost to me. Also, I know I will one day move here and live the rest of my life here. So what's four more years (or six+ with residency) outside of Israel?

But the problem is I feel like I've grown immensely this year as a person, and I'm not ready to give up that growth. Then again, medical school will be growth in a whole new spectrum of ways, that I've been hoping for forever. And being home in Montreal, I will be with the most important people in my life - my family. I miss them more than they know.

What is waiting for me at the end of each path, I can only guess. I hope the endings are the same, and that there is one destiny waiting for me that I can achieve either way. I must believe that, because right now I am about to call Ben Gurion and give up my place in next year's class.

Wish me luck.

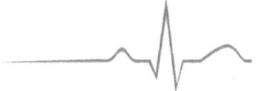

33

From Sorrow to Joy

<u>May 4, 2003</u>

Shalom,

I just got back from a *tiyul* to Tzfat, an ancient, beautiful hilltop city in the north of Israel. Being there was very refreshing, both physically and emotionally. In Jewish mystical tradition, Tzfat is the city of air — up on a mountaintop surrounded by sky and birds, one truly feels part of the realm of air. Jerusalem is the city of fire, because of *Aish Hakodesh* — the holy fire that often feels as if it is consuming one here. Tiberias is the city of water, as it is situated on Israel's prime water source - the Kinneret. Finally, Hevron is the city of earth; our forefathers and mothers are buried there.

I really felt the air quality of Tzfat, especially when we went hiking in Nachal Amud right outside the city. The path was in a riverbed, with steep cliffs on either side. I didn't need to use my ventolin (asthma medicine) the whole *tiyul* — not even on the incredibly long, steep ascent out of the canyon. We climbed straight up, sometimes hand and foot, over half a kilometre in order to exit the trail and meet our bus. My health truly feels miraculous, and I am thanking God for that every moment. As most of you know, my asthma has been excruciatingly difficult to deal with ever since my first attack in university - I even landed up in hospital one night here in Jerusalem. So not having to use ventolin at all for a period of days is unbelievable.

Hiking down a steep cliff outside Carmiel on Thursday, I had an experience that shook me up and taught me an important lesson. At any point in the descent, had I taken a wrong step, I would have fallen very far onto rocks, and throughout the hike there were immense numbers of thorn bushes pricking my legs. Halfway down I tripped (I still have no idea why) and fell, executing a quick roll and standing right back up all in one fluid motion. Everyone who saw me remarked on how gracefully I tumbled. I was fortunate not to have fallen far — I attribute that to my quick reflexes and also to someone "up there" looking out for me. As I began to walk again, I looked down and noticed my left arm was bleeding — turns out I had rolled through a thorn bush and had dozens of tiny thorns embedded in my arm, from palm to shoulder. Luckily, I was wearing jeans, so my legs were just bruised. However, my arm started stinging and burning, bleeding and swelling up. We took a break in the shade of a cave — ostensibly used by Elijah the prophet — and I started pulling myself together. We picked most of the thorns out and I cleaned up the wounds, and we continued on.

Later that day, I was thinking about why I would have fallen, and why into a thorn bush? I am not one to get hurt, have only broken one bone in my body (thumb during basketball) and hardly ever get sick. Plus, I have great balance. So why the fall? I concluded that it's possible that something much worse was supposed to happen to me on this *tiyul* — perhaps I was fated to fall farther, even die. Who knows? I'm thanking that thorn bush now, and whatever angel watches over me, for only giving me such negligible pain to deal with. I feel blessed to be in as good a condition as I am in physically. So thank God for thorns that prick, but do not kill. Just as Jews break a glass at a wedding, as the one bad thing that should ever happen in their marriage, so too should the thorn bush be in my life.

Tomorrow night *Yom Hazikaron* begins — Israel's memorial day commemorating her fallen soldiers. Following that, Tuesday night leads us into *Yom Ha'atzmaut* — Israel's Independence Day. My week is packed! Plus, my friend Gillian (from my time at Haifa MDA) arrives tonight, and my mother is coming in on Friday.

What a wonderful world.

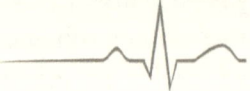

May 4, 2003

I'm sitting here outside Har Herzl, waiting for Yael and the rest of our MDA group.

There's a rehearsal of a *tekes* here tonight, the ceremony where we shift from *Yom Hazikaron* to *Yom Ha'atzmaut* — from sorrow to joy. Yael has tickets for us, so here I am!

It's really exciting to be here, a genuine part of Israeli society about to unfold before me. It feels amazing to find myself woven into the fabric of this country that I love.

How special to be here this week!

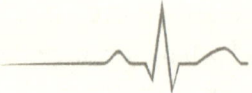

May 5, 2003

I am sitting in Kikar Rabin in Tel Aviv. This evening is *Yom Hazikaron*, and we came to this spot in order to listen to songs and the stories of soldiers and their families. We wanted to truly participate as a part of the people of Israel in the land of Israel. Now the song "Mah Avarech" is playing; before that we saw a quick clip of the Apter family, whose son was murdered in the *pigua* at the yeshiva in Otniel a few months ago.

This afternoon, after working at MDA, Gillian and I worked at a *Yom Hazikaron* ceremony at Yad Lebanim, where Ariel Sharon spoke. Then an army choir sang "Leorech Hayam", and we said Kaddish and El Maleh Rachamim, led by the chief rabbi of Tzahal (the IDF).

It is really special to be a part of this place, at this moment. I've been to three ceremonies already, with more over the next two days.

When we were driving here from Yerushalayim, there were memorials all along the highway; burned-out bunkers and army vehicles, lit by red lamps and draped with Israeli flags. The Azrieli towers here in Tel Aviv have incredibly long chains of flags hanging from them.

I am now standing at the spot where Yitzhak Rabin was killed. The flag is at half-mast.

On the way home, we'll go by Mike's Place, a bar that had a *pigua* last week, and light candles.

Lailah Tov.

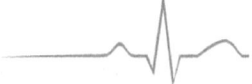

May 6, 2003

Yom Hazikaron

I am sitting in the military cemetery on Har Herzl, listening to Ariel Sharon speak. Gill and I broke off from the Pardes crowd to walk around with the Israelis, grieving with them in this place. There are thousands of people here. The siren blasted so loud that it cut a path for my tears, exploding my soul from within.

The *tekes* is over. I am sitting on stairs somewhere, watching my people, so many of them, move by me in comforting warm waves. Soldiers, family, kids, old people, Hebrew, Russian, English. Birds, cell phones, and under it all the constant rumble of thousands of voices. Now and then one voice comes into focus, then moves past and its spot in my consciousness is filled by another. But all are voices of my people, my person, extensions of my soul. I love them, alive and dead, with equal strength and passion.

Now leaving. Intense day. Need a corner to cry in.

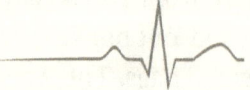

May 7, 2003

Last night *Yom Hazikaron* changed into *Yom Ha'atzmaut*, and we all went out to celebrate. Gill and I went to meet up with Yudah in Kikar Safra, outside the city hall on Jaffa Street. There was Israeli folk-dancing all night, and we tried to dance for a while. It was great; a few hundred people all doing *Rikudei Am*. At about midnight, we moved on to Ben Yehuda and got COVERED in shaving cream. It's such a strange *Yom Ha'atzmaut* tradition, people running around spraying shaving cream at strangers and bonking each other with plastic hammers. I wonder where it came from and why? I think part of it is being so free and happy with our Jewish state that for one night we can throw inhibition out the window and go crazy. There must have been ten thousand people in the streets!!

What a way to celebrate. I love this country.

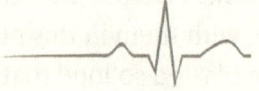

34

Smoke and Flames

May 19, 2003

Hi,

I'm exhausted, no time for a long email, five *piguim* in twenty-four hours.

Worked today, working tomorrow, working Wednesday and then Thursday night (on the ICU truck).

Didn't go to any of the bombings.

I'm safe, don't worry.

Will write when I have time.

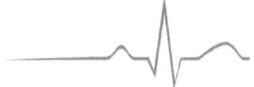

May 20, 2003: Lag Ba'Omer

This morning I'm working at MDA, as I did yesterday. I'm also working tomorrow a.m. and Thursday night.

Last night we celebrated Lag Ba'Omer, despite a rash of *piguim* (six in forty-eight hours). Fortunately, I wasn't at any of the attacks.

Last night was really fun; after work, I napped for an hour, then Gill and I went out.

First, we had a BBQ that started on the roof of Yudah's building but then moved to the park across the street. From the roof I could see smoke and flames rising on the horizons of the city, and while driving through Katamon at one point we saw Hasidim with tremendous bonfires. They had built two bonfires in the shape of teepees, probably about five metres tall, in a park. As we drove away, we could see fire rising above the roof of a building that separated us from the park. It reminded me of the descriptions of the Salem witch burnings. But, of course, the fires represent something completely different.

Lag Ba'Omer is the thirty-third day of counting the forty-nine days from Pesach to Shavuot. We celebrate because on this day Rabbi Akiva's students stopped dying (perhaps from a plague, about 24,000 of them). Bonfires are lit as reminiscent of the signal fires lit in those times on hilltops around Israel.

So last night Jerusalem was on fire, beautiful fire.

Barbecuing in the park on King George Street with Yudah, Aryeh, and the whole MDA crowd was really special. We ate *shipudim* (like kebabs) and sang songs for hours. At about midnight, a few of us headed over to a site near Sha'are Zedek Hospital, where the *Bnot Sherut* of MDA were having a bonfire. We hung out for a while, toasted marshmallows and relaxed. At various times ambulances would pull up to say hi, which was fun. At about 2:15, Gill and I got a ride with Ruti back to the station, where we slept about four hours. Now we're working. Couldn't ask for a better time.

This morning, the firefighters are racing around Jerusalem, extinguishing remaining fires. It's a wonder the city didn't burn to a crisp; I can't believe this ritual happens every year! But it was a fantastic night.

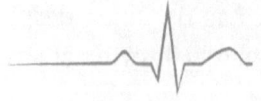

May 21, 2003

Thinking about things both before and after celebrating Lag Ba'Omer, I pondered how our country can party amid tragedy. After talking with Gill, I concluded that, like usual, Israel must not allow herself to become swallowed up by the fear all around her. We who live here must keep our lives going as normal (or almost normal) even in the face of incredible brutality and inconceivable massacres of innocents. When buses are blown up by eighteen-year-old boys and girls, there is not much one can do to come to terms with it.

Living here is living a very different type of existence than in Montreal. For instance, today I got an email about a memorial ceremony in Montreal for the victims of the six attacks we had in forty-eight hours. Memorials are great, but how useful are they, really? Yes, they unite us in our grief and they send a message of unity between the diaspora and Israeli Jews. But here in Israel, we formally memorialize our fallen once a year on *Yom Hazikaron*. On Har Herzl and in the other cemeteries around Israel, our people come to cry together, and support one another. On the day of a *pigua*, and for a day or two afterwards, the only thing on the news is that attack. We hear the names of the victims, see their faces and the faces of their families. We are told the times and places of their funerals in case we want to attend. And we unite in shock and sorrow. But then we pick ourselves up and move on with our lives here — as we must.

So on Lag Ba'omer, (here I break off to listen to a lot of sirens outside my window — did something happen?), we partied even through the anguish. But like Gill said when I discussed this with her, what makes this different and special is that through the celebration each Israeli carries in his or her mind and heart the memory and collective grief of a nation.

That is what makes Israel my home.

We share laughter and grief.

We share our stories, and our shared history.

There are those of us who see, as I do, hope dangling on a thin fishing line way off in the distant sea of future — and though we know we will not see it in our lifetimes, we cling to the promise of a God we first met thousands of years ago. A promise to live in a land flowing with milk and honey, an inheritance for our children and their children to eternity.

This is Israel.

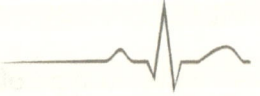

35

Prayers for Noa

May 22, 2003

Hi all,

My mom was here with me for a week and it was such a fantastic time. I really loved having Mom here to see my life and what I've built for myself. On the night Mom got in, I had a large Shabbat dinner with about sixteen of my closest friends. I thought she'd be overwhelmed, but she had a really great time, and my friends loved her, of course. Then we went to Shabbat lunch at Yudah's house with a whole different group of friends. She loved that, too.

We had a wonderful time, and I'm so proud of her, endlessly, for coming here, at this time, to visit Israel and me.

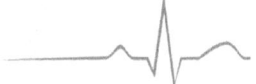

May 31, 2003

This week we celebrated *Yom Yerushalayim*, Jerusalem Day. On this day in 1967, Jerusalem's Old City was liberated and came into the folds of the Jewish State. During the evening my friends and I went to a free concert put on by Pardes in memory of two students, Marla Bennett and Ben Blutstein, who were killed in the bombing at Hebrew University last July 31. This concert took place on the Tayelet, a beautiful promenade overlooking all of Jerusalem, on a ridge that was the site of a few bloody battles to win this city. Sheva and Hadag Nahash played, two fantastic bands. I danced and sang in the middle of thousands of Israelis, young and old, and tourists. It was a perfect way to spend this important and celebratory night.

The next night Gillian and I worked an event-based shift on the ambulance, where we sat outside Mercaz HaRav (a *Dati Leumi* yeshiva) and watched all the yeshiva boys dance. We stayed there from 10:00 p.m. to 3:00 a.m., as dozens of people gave speeches. We listened to present and past chief rabbis including Rav Ovadia Yosef, along with Shaul Mofaz, Minister of Defense, Moshe Katzav, President of Israel, different Members of Knesset, the Chief Rabbi of Tzahal, and more. Finally at around 3:15, the crowd started moving off toward the Old City, and we followed behind them (there must have been at least 5000 people) in the ambulance until we arrived at the Kotel (Western Wall of the Temple) at about 4:45. We didn't get to bed till about 5:30 a.m.

It was a truly surreal experience for me to be standing at the Kotel on *Yom Yerushalayim*, wearing my Magen David Adom gear. The symbolism made me want to dance and sing, while at the same time collapse in a heap of tears for those who can't be here with us celebrating. My grandparents always wanted to see the Kotel, and I don't know if they ever got that chance. I thought to myself, and still think: here I am, in Jerusalem, standing at the base of a wall that so many of my ancestors never even got to see, and I am wearing a huge red Star of David emblazoned on my back and upon my heart. And no one is stopping me from being here, no one is shooting at the target my shirt makes. I am serving my free people in our free, strong, beautiful country, and I am living and working in the city which is the heart of our state. What a moment, what a year, what a life.

I feel so lucky and so blessed.

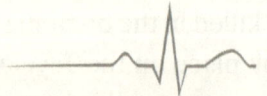

June 2, 2003

I just got back from a long, often stressful but overall wonderful day at Magen David Adom. Let me tell you about today, and about a baby girl whose tiny feet imprinted themselves upon my heart even though she cannot move them to do so.

Noa is ten months old and suffers from myotonic dystrophy, a musculoskeletal illness which prevents her from leading a normal baby life. She relies completely on others to breathe for her, feed her, clothe her, and move her. She lies in a baby hospital bed until she is stable enough to go home.

Today, our ambulance was called to transfer her from a pediatric intensive care unit to a different hospital. When we arrived at the PICU, I began communicating with Noa in whatever way one can with babies — touch, sound, facial expression. I smiled at her, gave her my gloved finger to grip, and watched her move her upper body around. She, unfortunately, didn't seem to have any movement in her lower body. The doctor and nurses were preparing Noa for transfer, but we realized what a severe case this was when the doctor said she had to come with us. Noa cannot breathe on her own, so the doctor had to bag her the whole ride (she had to give Noa breaths using a bag-valve-mask device). Everyone was occupied with the preparations, and I was the only one in the room who had my eye on Noa. Suddenly I noticed her face was getting slightly purple, her mouth was in an open *O*-shape and she was shaking her arms around. She was in obvious respiratory distress and needed suctioning and ventilation pronto. I began calling for the doctor, but no one was listening to me. I watched as her oxygen saturation fell from 100% to 83%, and by that time, I was almost screaming for the doctor. She finally came over, looking annoyed as hell, until she saw what was going on with Noa. Then two nurses and the doctor descended upon the baby and started suctioning and ventilating like crazy. My ambulance driver turned to me with a relieved look on her face, and said *Kol Hakavod*. I was just so happy that Noa didn't suffocate on her own secretions.

That moment really highlighted for me the need to become a doctor. I felt so helpless, standing over a choking baby and unable to intervene given my status in the hospital and my lack of knowledge apropos hospital protocol.

Besides reinforcing my commitment to medicine, specifically pediatric emergency medicine, the situation today kindled another fire inside of me. When I return to Canada at the beginning of August, I would like to begin speaking at venues about Magen David Adom. I want to fundraise for this incredible organization. We just do not have the resources we need to keep our country healthy and safe. Today our ambulance went out without a Lifepak (automated external defibrillator), because there weren't enough to go around! I cannot even imagine what would have happened if Noa had had a cardiac arrest in the ambulance, without a defibrillator present to restart her heart. To me and to the EMS world, it must be completely unacceptable to proceed with such a lack of equipment. Magen David Adom needs money, and we need equipment. I am ready to come back to Canada and work like mad to get the funds. I hope that all of you reading this letter will be interested in this idea, and can spread the word. I want to raise money in a specific way, directed to specific equipment. I haven't begun the process yet, but I am brainstorming. If you have any ideas, please let me know.

For now, please direct any prayers you have in you toward Noa, that she be able to lead a somewhat normal life one day. Or at least, that she shouldn't suffer.

P.S. I'll be working tonight from 11 to 7, tomorrow 3 p.m. to 7 a.m. in Haifa, and Wednesday 11 to 7 in Haifa. See you on the other side of exhaustion.

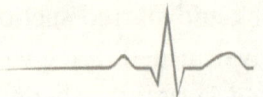

36

Time Stops

June 11, 2003

Hello,

I'm about to go to bed. It's 2:30 a.m. here, but I feel an intense obligation to let you all know that I am fine.

There was a huge bombing in the heart of Jerusalem today; a Palestinian suicide bomber, dressed like an Ultra-Orthodox Jew, blew up bus no.14. He carried an enormous bomb full of metal fragments that subsequently did a lot of damage.

I will write a whole long email maybe tomorrow night, but for now know this much: I was at Magen David Adom, in the bathroom after a long shift, when the siren sounded and the call came over the speakers for all drivers to get to the ambulances. I ran out to my driver, Dudu's, ambulance, #60, and we took off with two other guys. We were the fourth or fifth ambulance on-scene, and since we only had two shrapnel-proof vests, Dudu had me stay by the ambulance and guard it with my life till he came back. We guard the ambulances because a *pigua* is the perfect time for a terrorist to steal one for later use, and also because only the driver of that specific ambulance should take it from the chaotic scene.

To make a long story short for now, I bagged (ventilated) one patient for a while until we realized there was no saving him, and then we took a moderately injured patient to one of the hospitals. By the end, our ambulance was covered in pools of blood; my clothes are covered as I sat in the blood, and even after a long shower I still smell blood on me.

I have so much more to say, but I'm in no proper emotional state to sit here and type. Just know that I am alive, and hopefully everyone I know here is alive — but sixteen people are murdered, eighty people are injured and everyone connected, even remotely, to this *pigua* is scarred for life and suffering. I am in intense agony inside, but we had a two hour debriefing at MDA and my friends are here for me. So I will be ok. Please do me a favour — send a prayer or wish or hope or whatever to whomever or whatever you choose and ask in it that peace should come to this place. Ask for an end to these bombings, ask for mercy on the innocent people that suffer. Ask for health for the patients still in hospital, for their families and for all of us who were there at the scene — we also need you.

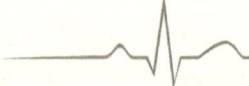

Friday, June 13, 2003

Two days after the *pigua* on Rechov Yafo here in Jerusalem, on June 11 at 5:30 p.m.

It's very important that I write down everything from that day and onwards — what happened, how I felt and feel, what I did, etc, because this event is hitting me much harder than the last *pigua* I worked at.

Wednesday started out a very boring, routine day. I got on an ambulance with Zohar, a driver that I've been crushing on. I was very excited, but then two hours later he was transferred to the *Natan* and I joined Benji's ambulance. Benji is young, handsome and Israeli American; he wants to be a doctor one day so we have a lot to talk about. He is married to a wonderful woman named Malka, who is kind and supportive. I work as often with Benji as I do with Dudu, and every time is a lot of fun. We spent the whole day Wednesday playing cards with a few other people, because there were no calls. It was a completely quiet day, and at the end of my shift I went for burgers with some friends then joined Dudu's ambulance. We had one call, a hard one though. We took a seventeen-year-old boy who had fallen off a horse and had a severe head injury. He couldn't speak to me because his mouth was full of blood, but he was alert and we were able to communicate through hand squeezes.

When we got back to the station, I went to the bathroom while Dudu went to park the ambulance. Suddenly, with my pants around my ankles, I heard an incredibly loud and unmistakable beeping noise from the loudspeakers, followed by the call for all drivers to go to the ambulances. I ran out of the washroom, still doing up my belt, into absolute mayhem. Everyone present in the station was hurtling toward the ambulances. Through the chaos I glimpsed #60, Dudu's ambulance, and dove in through the side door. There were three of us plus Dudu, and he took off while barking orders to put on the flak vests. Others kept trying to get in the ambulance, but Dudu kicked them off because the maximum crew is supposed to be four. There were only two flak vests — no ambulance has more than that — so Dudu and the guy in the front put them on. Dudu told me and the other guy that we would have to stay by the ambulance without flak vests, because it's just not safe (terrorists have been known to plant a second, and even sometimes a third bomb, to detonate upon arrival of the ambulances).

Our ambulance flew down the street, past the central bus station, and right into downtown Jerusalem. Suddenly, ahead of us loomed the smoking carcass of the bus, #14-aleph, which was my usual bus route. Thank God I only found out which line it was after I dropped off my patient. Had I known earlier, I would have really been in shock. I ride that bus almost every day, and often at that exact time of day. Had I been back at the station earlier and caught the usual bus home, I may have been a casualty instead of a rescuer.

The scene was insane; people running everywhere, screaming, police and medics trying to get the situation under control... Ambulances in front of us, ambulances behind us, a long line of lights and sirens and foreboding. In the midst of it all, the patients... the bystanders... the bright June sunshine and surrealistic feeling of being in a movie. Dudu and both of the other guys jumped off, and I threw the backboard on the bed with a collar and the ambu bag (resuscitation equipment). I was so calm; time felt like it was standing still. I went through all the motions that I knew needed to be done, and then Dudu was beside me, telling me to guard the ambulance with my life. He ran off with the bed and equipment, leaving me to wait and prepare the ambulance.

By the time the first patient came to me (about thirty seconds that felt like a year), I was ready. Looking around me, I saw more ambulances pulling up. Tzuri was beside our ambulance and I watched coolly as two medics ran around the back of his ambulance with a bed. They almost got hit as he backed up, but they continued running down the hill toward the bus. They were so out of control that their bed fell over and one of them fell as well. I wanted to go over and say, calm down, you can't treat patients when you're under such *lachatz*. You need to keep your cool or you won't do anyone any good.

I can see this footage in my head, like a scene from TV: two people in orange medic vests came running at me from the bus, pulling a bed with a man on it. When they got to me, we assessed his vitals; his eyes were wide open, fixed and dilated, he wasn't breathing but he had a pulse. Someone had already inserted an orange airway into his mouth. The medics started to load him on the ambulance, but I told them I was waiting for my driver to bring patients. I leaned over and closed the patient's eyes, but they popped back open (reflex, I suppose, because he wasn't responding at all). The medics put him on the ambulance anyway, and one of them (a volunteer driver, apparently) started trying to drive off. Thank goodness Dudu got there in time and stopped them; he had another patient on a backboard. Meanwhile, I was in the back alone with the patient, and I had begun bagging him as soon as he was in the back with me. But his chest wasn't rising, even though I tried repeatedly to open his airway with a head tilt/chin lift. After what felt like forever but was probably only a couple of minutes, Dudu came in the back with me and told me to stop because the man would not survive. He had apparently lost his pulse. We took him off the ambulance and loaded the other patient instead, and as the bed was rolling out the back doors, I could see a vast pool of blood all over the floor of the ambulance. The patient had obviously bled out and there was nothing we could do for him.

I have to stop for a moment and explain the multi-casualty incident and how it differs from regular treatment of patients. In an *Aran* such as a bombing, we try to save those people that have a chance of survival ahead of those that may not make it. There is a triage system, using a colour code, so that we medics make sure to transport those who have a reasonable chance of survival. My non-breathing patient had suffered such traumatic bodily injuries that saving him was probably impossible; he had probably already suffered irreversible brain damage as well. On the other hand, the patient we ended up transporting is still alive (although undergoing operations).

Ariel is a twenty-year-old MDA medic who right now is lying in the recovery room at Hadassah Ein Karem Hospital after back surgery. When Dudu loaded him into the ambulance, I immediately started talking to him and checking his injuries. The first thing he said to me was "I forgot my medic kit on the bus!" followed quickly by "Who is *Pikud Eser?*". The first thing I noticed about Ariel was his face: big green eyes with golden-brown flecks, curly blondish hair (turns out he actually has straight, short dark hair...), and a big puncture wound on his right cheek where a piece of metal or a nail had entered his body. Through a full-body check, I found a hole in his upper left chest by the clavicle, and another one in his inner right thigh by the pelvis. We cut off all of his clothes, and I found that his entire genital area was soaked in blood; I still don't know from what. There was already a bandage on his thigh, and I asked Dudu if I should put an Ascherman Chest Seal on the chest wound. Dudu decided it wasn't necessary, so I just monitored the injuries, took Ariel's vital signs and information, and talked to him the entire ride to Shaare Zedek Hospital. He was terrified, and he wanted me to call his mom using his cell phone. I tried a few times, but to no avail - the whole cell phone network goes down during a *pigua* because often there is another terrorist who needs the cell network to detonate a bomb.

When we arrived at Shaare Zedek, there were dozens of people waiting for us; within seconds of opening our doors, doctors and nurses were helping us unload Ariel. There were tons of news cameras and journalists behind the crowds of medical personnel. Dudu and I ran in the doors to the ER just like you see in a scene from *ER* the TV show. It was surreal. We ran into the crash room with Ariel, where they started working on him right away. I pushed myself up against the wall, trying to stay out of the way while Dudu filled out the MCI card with the patient's info on it. A nurse called to me to come help as they inserted a catheter; Ariel was screaming and struggling, and I had to help hold him down. I called to him to let him know it would be okay, but to no avail. After about five minutes, Dudu and I left, and once outside, the situation began to hit me.

I remember being in the ambulance and looking down to see my glove torn open on the palm, then hastily switching gloves. I remember the awful sweet smell of blood, in the ambulance, on my clothes, all over me. Sitting in the dead man's blood to treat Ariel, blood on my pants and shirt, hands and shoes. Blood everywhere. I remember going down Ariel's body with my gloved hands, and feeling slivers of glass and metal trying to penetrate me as well.

After leaving the ER, we stood outside by the ambulance and I called Mom, got a call from Nadav and Chen, and started to clean up. The whole time I was cleaning garbage from inside the ambulance, I couldn't stop singing "Biglal Haruah" and "Yihyeh Tov" — I just couldn't stop singing. It was sick, but I suppose my mind's reaction to such severe trauma.

Dudu came up to me as I was standing outside the ambulance, and he put his arm around me. He told me that I had done a good job, and that he was proud of me. He emphasized how happy he was that our ambulance came out unscathed, and with almost all of our equipment (apparently many ambulances get ransacked for equipment at the site of a *pigua*, by people needing to treat quickly). This was the first time that Dudu really showed me affection, and I really needed it at that moment. He is kind of my mentor here, at least that's how I consider him, and it felt reassuring to have his arm around me at that moment. It was also extremely important to me to hear that I had done a good job, because when a patient dies on you, you always wonder what you could have done to save him. Dudu repeatedly told me that there was nothing I could have done.

When we got back to the station, we went to wash down the ambulance. We removed all the bloody equipment, bed, backboard, ambu, etc, and I washed them down outside the ambulance. Dudu, in the meantime, hosed down the inside of the ambulance, and the bench which was bloody. It took us a little while. Time again felt like it was standing still as I carefully wiped all the blood off the equipment. At that point, I noticed my arms were covered in blood, all the way up the forearm, and that it had dried already. I didn't make any effort to wash it off until a couple of hours later... it just didn't feel like a priority.

I spent the next little while waiting for everyone to get back to the station. As my friends pulled up in various ambulances, we all came over to greet each other, but we were all, naturally, very subdued. I stood near the entrance to Beit HaMitnadev and watched a particularly beautiful orange-red sunset; now that I think about it, it looked like a painting made of the blood I cleaned up.

At about 8 p.m. we had a debriefing session with everyone who had worked the *pigua*. Obviously, not everyone came, but there were probably about a hundred people there. The heads of MDA and the Jerusalem station, including the chief paramedic etc., broke down the event for us with diagrams and summaries. Then, each driver was asked to describe how many patients they had transported, their injuries, etc. When it was Dudu's turn, he told them about both our patients, and then someone asked who had worked with him. So he put his hand on my shoulder and motioned to me and one of the other medics that had come with us. It felt strange to be singled out in the MDA crowd.

After the debriefing, many people left but I just couldn't get up the *koach* to leave my friends. I was waiting for Yael and Yudah and the rest of the crowd to show up and talk things out with me, when a volunteer driver named Shlomi got a call. He had no one with him in the ambulance, so I went even though I really didn't want to. We pulled up to a scene almost as chaotic as the *pigua*; a car accident, bus vs taxi. A *Natan* truck was already there, and as I came up from our ambulance with equipment,

Erez (a freckle-faced, red-headed paramedic) stopped me. He put his hand on my shoulder, then on my cheek, and held my face while asking me how I felt and if I was OK to work. In that moment, time stopped, and I felt sobbing welling up inside of me. All the pain of the day threatened to break over us like Niagara Falls, but I held it together. I told him I was OK, and thanked him, and we went to treat the patients.

The scene was a mess; dozens of Haredi men and boys standing and gawking. I had to push my way through them forcibly with the equipment - they just didn't get it! They drove me crazy. I hate when people stand around gawking at someone else's pain.

We finally loaded two badly injured Haredi male patients into the ambulance, and Shlomi was in the driver's seat right away while I began to treat. But five or six Haredim and Konnanim were making such a *balagan* trying to climb in the ambulance and yelling orders, that I couldn't do anything. Finally, I stopped and said "stop with this chaos! Everyone OFF the ambulance now!" They all left except for one guy who sat in the front seat to come with us, and he tried to come in the back with me. I told him to stay where he was because there was no place for him to sit in the back, what with two severely injured patients and me. Meanwhile, I was treating these men as per protocol, and doing a damn good job of it if I do say so myself, considering the stress. But then, as we were driving with lights and sirens, and I was administering oxygen and trying to assess further injuries, the patients started refusing treatment. They decided that since I am a woman, I couldn't touch them. Can you believe it? Someone with a head injury, chest injury, abdominal injury etc., refusing treatment based on the sex of the medic? So I said to them, "Look, I'm the only medic in the back of the ambulance with you, and I am THE medic here. I am treating you, and if you don't want that, then there's no one else to do it instead of me." So I continued with the treatment, and at one point the oxygen mask fell off one of them on a sharp turn. He immediately started yelling that this is what happens when a woman treats people. Finally, I was so sick of their stupid shtick that I said "Look, I worked at a *pigua* today. I don't want to hear any more of this shtick. We're going to the hospital and you'll be treated there, and I am so sorry that I am a woman." (Heavy on the sarcasm there.)

What a pain in the ass, I have to say, especially after a *pigua*. But I learned how tough I really can be, and how much I can put my foot down. I also learned that people can be really stupid.

OK, enough for now. Must go to sleep, though time feels like it's hit the pause button.

Will life ever be the same?

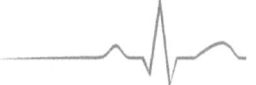

37

Sunshine, Chaos, Rainbows, Darkness

June 18, 2003

Hi all,

Some incredible news.... the guy that I brought in from the *pigua*, who is a volunteer at Magen David Adom, woke up this morning after being under anaesthesia for a week. He had a few operations, but it seems that he's going to be just fine! I feel incredible, like I really saved a life — Dudu and I saved a life. This young man is going to have the rest of his life to live, thankfully, with scars both external and internal, but at least he's got another chance. I can't tell you how amazing this makes me feel. When I heard that he had woken up, I almost started crying. I am still on the verge of tears. I have been crying all week on and off, but these tears are of joy rather than sorrow, so they feel totally different.

Now, after that wonderfully refreshing story of actual survival, let me move on to a darker story. Sorry to have to go back to such things, but that's the reality of life in this country: sunshine followed by chaos followed by rainbows followed by blackness.

Yesterday morning I worked a shift with a driver I love, Boaz, and two other medics. Boaz is a tall, lanky, silly, wonderful man, who lives with his wife and young daughter on the outskirts of Jerusalem. Along with working as an ambulance driver and medic, Boaz works in the stocking room at MDA Jerusalem. Working with him is always fun; he blasts Israeli contemporary music and makes me laugh. We have a really great friendship. Boaz has been working for MDA for a while, and two years ago he survived the firebombing of his ambulance at the start of the second intifada — in fact, Dudu rescued him.

Yesterday, dispatch sent us to an Arab school in Ras al-Amud, an Arab neighbourhood in East Jerusalem, to help a sick teacher. We had a *livui*, but it didn't seem to be an out of the ordinary call (we get escorted every time we go into an Arab area). We drove down a steep, narrow drive into the school's tiny parking lot, between the building and an enclosed playground. On getting out of the ambulance, a din so loud you could hardly hear yourself think immediately surrounded us. All the kids in the school were yelling at us, standing at the windows and banging on the bars, throwing garbage at us. Outside, there were about twenty little boys running around us with sticks and steel bars, but there were teachers and older students chasing them back inside (not that they were very successful).

Boaz turned to us and told us to stand with our backs to the school wall while he turned the ambulance around so we could have a quick exit. Guarding us was a border policeman with a nice big gun. I was getting pelted with garbage — it was getting quite scary there. Finally, Boaz came back, and we all went to get the teacher around the back of the school. As we were climbing the stairs to get her, Boaz turned to us and said, "When we leave, Sara goes in the middle of a circle that we'll make around her (he and the other two male medics), because we all have handguns except her." Imagine how I felt at that moment. But when we got back outside, Boaz decided to place two of the Arab teachers in our midst to help us, so that it would deter the kids from hurting us. We made it back no problem, loaded her on, and started to leave. As we pulled out, the kids were hurling stones at the ambulance, but only managed to hit the army jeep behind us as we sped out of there.

Listen, before yesterday I knew the phrase "hatred from birth", and I was fully aware of the fact that some Arab kids here are taught to hate, fear and want to kill the Jews. But I never ever fully understood what that meant. I never digested the fact that, yes, little children would kill me if they could. My idealistic soul always held on to the catchphrase "look for the good in everyone". Well, how can I look for good when I come to do a good deed and help someone in need, only to get pelted with garbage and rocks? Never mind the names those kids were calling me — the words in Arabic are so close to Hebrew that I knew exactly what they were saying.

Now I understand. Now I am even more afraid for this tiny nation of ours, and now I am even more sure that peace is a long way away (if possible at all).

I haven't lost hope - but I stared hate and death in the face, and the face was that of a six-year-old child in a schoolyard in Ras al-Amud.

Wish for peace.

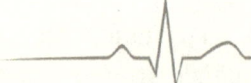

June 19, 2003

Hey all,

I wanted to share some great news. I went to visit Ariel in the ICU today, the patient I brought from the *pigua*. Dudu and I went together, and it was a really pleasant visit. There was another MDA girl there visiting him. When we walked into the ICU, he immediately recognized us and waved. We went over and started talking with him; he had to communicate with hand motions because his face is all swollen from jaw surgery. He looks pretty messed up, all bruised and swollen, but to me the yellow under his right eye is sunshine. It means he is alive, and that is all that matters.

I noticed the card that I had brought him while he was still unconscious — it was sitting on a shelf by the bed. I gave it to him, and he read it right there and then. He gave me a big thumbs up and tried to smile. I almost cried.

Before Dudu and I left, we wished him *Refuah Shlemah* and I told him I can't wait to see him at MDA again soon. We shook his hand to say goodbye — he had a good firm grip — and left. I am so happy. It's like floating on clouds to know that he survived and will go on with his life. I just wish the same for all the injured.

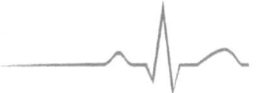

38

Death, Birth, Death, Birth

June 29, 2003

The year at Pardes is over, and I am moving out of this apartment here on Rivka Street, tomorrow evening after work. My roommates have already left, and I am the last one here. Today I am spending my whole day cleaning and packing, trying to make this place spotless, so I get my whole security deposit back. Tomorrow my internet is being disconnected, and this laptop is spending the month at a friend's apartment given that I am moving to the new immigrant absorption center (not the most secure place for valuables). The Jewish Agency, who arranged and funded my internship this year at MDA, is paying for me to stay at the absorption center. I will try to get online a few times each week, but no promises. Please continue emailing me, but avoid sending large files because my hotmail will crash.

I'm always reachable on my cell phone. But remember that if, God forbid, another *pigua* happens, don't call me right away. I won't be able to answer the phone if the *pigua* is in Jerusalem, because I'll be working. Call me about an hour after, and I'll be able to take the call. This goes for everyone except my parents and sisters. You guys can call me right away, and if possible, I'll take the phone.

Miss you all; see you in a month.

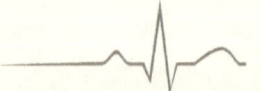

June 30, 2003

Just moved out of my apartment on Rivka Street. Now I'm sitting in my newly set-up room at Beit Canada, the immigrant absorption center here in Jerusalem. It's pretty nice actually, but I will be sharing one bedroom with two other women when they arrive (probably by next week). For now, I've got the place to myself, which is nice, albeit a teensy bit lonely. Oh well, I'd better get used to being alone in an apartment.

I've got to go to bed soon, I'm working at MDA at 7 a.m. and it's already 1 a.m... Gotta leave here by 6.

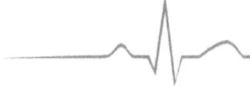

July 3, 2003

I'm sitting in my room in Beit Canada. I still have the place to myself, which is great; last night one girl slept here, but they moved her to a different room today. I'm actually not just sitting, I'm hiding out from an enormous and scary hornet that is right now dashing its brains out against the light in my entranceway. I can't, for the life of me, figure out how to make it leave; it was hard enough getting it out of my bedroom! Going back and forth to the bathroom will be intense during the night... intensely frightening! Not only am I deathly afraid of bees, wasps and hornets, I am deathly allergic.

On to the next topic... since I have many to write up tonight and not that much energy.

A couple of days ago (Tuesday, July 1) I participated in my first full CPR. I say "first full CPR" because at the *pigua* on June 11, I performed artificial respirations on one man who subsequently died. On Tuesday, I was working with Dudu and our first call of the day was an errand. On the way, another ambulance was called to a CPR at the dialysis unit of Bikur Cholim Hospital, but we happened to be right next to it. So Dudu called in that we would take the call, and in we went.

We came to the scene of a sixty-five-year-old woman in cardiac arrest, with doctors and nurses performing CPR with the patient on a soft, pliable bed! They had been doing likely ineffective compressions for several minutes before we arrived. After four minutes of lack of oxygen to the brain, a person has irreversible brain damage. And without effective compressions, she wasn't getting any oxygen to her brain. The first thing we did was move her onto the floor, where Dudu began compressions with the cardiopump, and the *mishtalem nehigah* began giving breaths with the ambu. I took out all the equipment, began suctioning her as she brought up blood and mucus, and did whatever else needed to be done. Dudu and I had to correct the other medic many times; he wasn't holding the head back effectively enough to maintain a good airway, and he was exerting too much pressure too forcefully on the ambu. Her stomach started to inflate with air because of this. Anyway, after a few minutes that felt like forever, the *Natan* arrived with paramedics and a doctor. They jumped in with us and had me exert pressure on the patient's stomach to take out the air. Erez intubated the woman, and they started an IV. They tried adrenaline and atropine as well. The good news in all of this is that when the doctor checked the patient's pulse, she told us it had come back (albeit weakly). So we performed a semi-successful CPR (she died later in the hospital).

The act of performing CPR on someone should be something that would hit me harder than it did, I think. I first learned resuscitation (artificial respiration) at the age of eight, in swim classes, and learned CPR a few years later. So I've been practicing this for more than half my life, and during university I taught CPR for years. When we were helping our patient, I felt as if it was just another practice run — I knew exactly what to do, when, and how. I was comfortable in the situation, totally calm, just running down the checklist in my head of what to do. The situation didn't freak me out at all, to tell the truth. I suppose I'll make a good ER doc.

Today I assisted at another birth. Death, birth, death, birth... one continual cycle that I now feel truly a part of. A death and a birth in two days; this is only the beginning of what my life as a doctor will be like. Just a taste.

Working with Boaz today was a real treat. I adore being on his ambulance, and just being around him makes me smile. He's a good guy, and a great medic. He asked me to work with him on Tuesday, but I was working with Dudu. So we worked together today — and what a day to choose!

On our last call of the day, they sent us out halfway to Beit Shemesh to pick up a *yoledet* from the Beit Shemesh *Natan* truck. Boaz knew I'd helped deliver two babies already, so he put me down at the delivery end while he drove as fast as possible to the hospital. I was proud of myself for being ready for it - the *Bat Sherut*, Ayalah, was originally in that spot, but wasn't sure she could handle it. Boaz asked me, and I said I hadn't delivered a baby on my own but that I could definitely do it. So I sat by the delivery end of this pretty twenty-year-old Ethiopian woman and waited. Her contractions were still about two minutes apart, and I didn't think she would give birth in the ambulance. Her water broke, and I could see things moving inside of her. The head wasn't coming out yet though, so I knew we'd get her to the hospital on time.

Once in the delivery room, Boaz let me stay and watch the birth. He told me I had done a great job in the ambulance, which is a fantastic compliment coming from an MDA driver. Within about five to ten minutes, the woman gave birth to a baby girl. It was a difficult delivery, however, and I'm glad I didn't have to do it. Her head came out, went back in, came out, went back in, over and over. The doctor finally took hold of the head and was pulling it, which really upset me because I've always learned to pull the baby out by the shoulders. The head was coming out egg-shaped, really distorted looking, and totally bluish-purple. I could see the face coming out slowly underneath, facing downward, and it took a while before it came out in its entirety. At that point of pulling on the baby's head and neck, the doctor realized the cord was wrapped around the neck twice. She unraveled it and finally got the baby out. The doctor immediately put her down on the bed and clamped the cord slowly. She didn't suction out the mouth and nose, just picked the baby up by her ankles and started slapping her on the soles of her feet. She rubbed her back and shook her a bit, and part of the time didn't even notice that the baby's head was scrunched onto the bed. I was so frustrated, and wanted to take the baby and suction her so she would breathe!! Finally, she made a small noise, and she opened her eyes and looked at me. I was the first person to say "shalom, baby!" The doctor took her to a table and worked on her for a bit until we heard the healthy crying. I stayed and talked to the new mom while this was going on, because no one was with her; they just left her there exposed to the world!

Never ever let anyone take me to give birth at Bikur Cholim!

Anyway... so that was birth #3 this year. Boaz gave me a clamp for my bag (where I collect unused plastic clamps from each birth — the ones we use to clamp the cord). I now have a fine collection running down the spine of the bag, next to the patches of the countries I visited in Europe.

Things at MDA are going so well. Drivers now ask me to work with them, instead of vice versa, and I get along so well with everyone. Even people I've never worked with (i.e., cute paramedics) say hi and stop to chat with me. It's great; some people even think I'm Israeli. If I wasn't going to start McGill medical school, I would never leave this place. At least I know I'm going to come back each summer, and make aliyah ASAP. But leaving in a month will be hell. I really feel like my life is here now. Nevertheless, I also realize what a blessing it is to get into McGill; it's my life's dream. I've been wanting this for so long! I owe it to myself to do this, and I owe it to Israel and my future children. In terms of Israel, I know I can better serve this country and her people as a doctor. For my children, I know they deserve a mother with a stable and profitable career that she is happy and satisfied with. For myself — I would never forgive myself if I didn't go to McGill medical school now that I was accepted.

OK, I have more to write but must go to sleep; heading to Efrat this Shabbat, and staying at the home of one of my favourite drivers, Sabin.

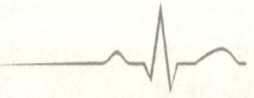

July 11, 2003

Shabbat Shalom!

Well, I've finally made it to the internet cafe and so I'm sending out what I hope will be a brief email. I'm having a great time at MDA as usual, working all the time and hardly eating or sleeping. For me, that's the way to live right now; I need to keep busy so I don't dwell on the horrible fact that I have to leave this wonderful country in seventeen days.

Last Shabbat, I spent the weekend at Sabin's home in Efrat — she's one of my favourite ambulance drivers. Shlomit, another driver that I love, also lives in Efrat with her family, and she and Sabin are best friends. They are really the cutest: two short, kind, matronly women who treat me like a little sister. We had dinner on Friday at Sabin's, and lunch on Saturday at Shlomit's. Between them, they have seven fun kids between the ages of five and eleven. Shlomit then invited me to stay with her until I leave Israel, but Efrat is twenty minutes outside Jerusalem in the Judean hills (West Bank). I would have to take a bulletproof bus every morning at about 6 to get to work on time... not the best idea. Efrat is a beautiful settlement (really more like a town, with 1800 families); to one side of it is Neve Daniel, and on another hill is Elazar. Behind Elazar is Alon Shvut. This area is called Gush Etzion, and it is a remarkable place to visit (despite the fact that Bet Lechem is right next door).

Two days ago, the MDA overseas volunteers program asked me to take a group of volunteers up to the Acre-Naharia area, almost at the Lebanese border. It's the first time we've sent volunteers up there, so the program coordinators wanted to make sure they got settled in appropriately. In this newest course of volunteers we have seventy-two people from all over the world! When we arrived in Naharia, I helped the group (five guys, nineteen to twenty-six-years-old, one French, on Brit, one American and two Canadians) move into their absorption center. It is located right on the beach, and it is full of Ethiopian and South American new immigrants. What an experience, even for one night! We had a fantastic time. After moving in and getting everything settled, we went into "town" (really just one long strip of restaurants) and had some food. Then we sat on the beach under the stars with beer and *nargila*, until about 1:30 a.m. At one point I looked up and saw a blazing shooting star that lasted a good three seconds, and then ten minutes later, three men galloped by on horseback down the beach. It was surreal.

The next morning, I took the guys to the Acre station, where a group of youth volunteers greeted us. They had come early in the morning because they were so excited to meet foreign volunteers! They made us feel so welcome, and the volunteer coordinator there was fantastic. All in all, I had a great time.

On the train back toward Jerusalem, I sat among what felt like a thousand soldiers all going home for Shabbat - a truly Israeli moment. A really old man came and sat down next to some soldiers, dressed in a Mexican outfit, and played the accordion. It was a lot of fun.

Finally, the other day, Ariel, the guy that Dudu and I saved from the *pigua*, came to visit at MDA. It was amazing to see him, hug him, chat with him for a while. It's an incredible experience to become friendly with someone whose life you helped to prolong. I am so happy that he is alive and doing so well.

I miss you all!!

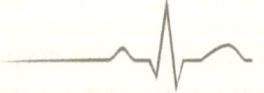

39

Terrorist Transport

<u>July 21, 2003</u>

Yesterday I worked the evening shift with my friends Judy and Dena (Judy is from Montreal, and Dena is from the US — they are both lovely girls that I've been fortunate enough to get to know well this year). In the middle of the shift, my driver was called to the *Moked* and then came outside to ask us whether we were comfortable taking a certain call. Turns out they tasked us with transporting a terrorist from a Jerusalem hospital to a military prison hospital about an hour away. We took five minutes to talk it over amongst ourselves. We had to consider seriously the fact that he was a terrorist and that we would have to be on the road at least two hours round-trip. The driver, my friend Benji, didn't want to give this man the pleasure of "looking at three pretty girls" the entire ride to jail, and none of us felt good about transporting a man who might hurt us if he had the chance. In the end, curiosity and itching to go out on a call, any call, took over, and we set out on the condition that there would be soldiers in the ambulance with us.

On the way to the hospital, my mind and heart swam with a whole sea of emotions, from anger to fear, from curiosity to nausea. I knew that at some point in my time here in Israel I would have to confront the question of: Do you treat a terrorist? If you treat a terrorist, how do you treat him? What do you do? What do you say? Do you come at the situation unbiased, as one is trained to do in medicine, or is it understandable if emotion comes into play? Do you talk to him as you talk to other patients, comfort him, try to ease his pain? Do we reserve the judgement for the judges and the ultimate Judge? How? Is he still human? If I chose not to treat him, would that make me therefore less human?

During my medical school interviews they asked me that overarching ethical question, "What would you do if you were faced with a wounded terrorist and he was in your care?" I answered the same way my heart answered in the actual confrontation with reality. I answered that I would treat him as I would treat any human being. But I would employ a system of "moral triage", a term I invented to explain the following concept. If I were to arrive at the scene of a terrorist incident and be faced with a wounded terrorist, I would first treat the victims. Once all the victims were adequately cared for, only then would I turn to the terrorist and dress his wounds. But there is no question in my heart and soul that I would treat him; who am I to judge him? Even though I may know that he just killed people, my people, I know it is only right to continue being human. By not treating him, I would essentially sink to his level and potentially become a killer myself. I truly believe that when someone is suffering, no matter who that person is, it is only right to help them and reserve judgement for later. And now all these things I am saying are no longer just theoretical; I cannot say to myself "well, you say one thing now but wait till the actual situation arises!" The theoretical is no longer just that; it has become factual.

We entered the patient's room to find a young man, perfectly normal looking except with a big dressing on his leg and three soldiers from the military police guarding him. He did not look evil, and even knowing what he did couldn't convince me that he was evil. I would really like to tell you who this man was, and what he did, but because of confidentiality and security issues, I am not allowed to reveal any such information. Suffice it to say that he did not kill anyone, or even physically injure anyone. But he committed a serious act of terrorism with large ramification for victim and country, and was potentially planning worse.

They handcuffed the prisoner's hands and feet, and the soldiers sat on the bench alongside him with their M-16s. Judy sat in front, I sat in the paramedic chair, and Dena sat at the end of the bench closest to me. In this way, the terrorist couldn't see us, and we didn't have to look at him. Because the call was just a transport and he didn't need any treatment,

I felt fine with the seating arrangement. Had he needed monitoring, I would have sat on the bench alongside him, terrorist or not.

I have to say, the ambulance ride itself was really fun. As sick as that sounds, I suppose it is the Israeli way of getting through hard situations. Just as the police at the Kiryat Menachem *pigua* flirted with me as I washed the cuts on their hands, so did these soldiers chit-chat with us the entire ride. We had a great time talking to these guys, who were aged twenty-one to twenty-three. After about forty-five minutes, we got to the prison, where we girls had to wait outside with one soldier while the ambulance continued inside. The soldiers had to leave their guns at the entrance with the guard, which scared me a bit. Even the soldier guarding us had to give up his rifle. We waited for thirty minutes outside, and a prisoner who was doing maintenance flirted it up with Dena. Then the prison security guards drove by repeatedly, and would stop and flirt with us. Having been in an Israeli prison before with the ambulance (in Haifa), I knew what to expect and just ignored all these guys; they were repulsive. Finally, the driver and the other soldiers reappeared in the ambulance. We took some pictures outside the jail and drove to get dinner. We had another fun ride back to Jerusalem, talking and laughing the whole time. Finally, we dropped them at the base.

What a night. I am glad we took the call, because now I know that I have no qualms about treating all manner of persons. Yes, it is difficult to think about helping a man who in another situation might kill you or your loved ones. But in reality, when I was faced with the human being, flesh and blood, the fact that he was a terrorist and enemy to all I hold dear took a back seat to my instinct to treat.

Listen, there is much more to the whole situation than I have described here so far. Many more thoughts ran through my head, and Judy, Dena, Benji and I talked for a while about what we felt throughout the ride. Having a Palestinian terrorist in such close proximity to me made me consider the cause they are fighting for. Had the man beside me been a suicide bomber or a man who had killed my people, I don't know if these thoughts would have come to me. But since he had not even actually physically injured a person, and didn't seem to be a blood-lusting murderer, my thoughts ran freely toward understanding him. I saw a frustrated guy, upset at the situation his people are in, fed hatred from the cradle, and living in a place of terrorism. No doubt he had friends who blew themselves up in order to kill Israelis. He must have felt intense pressure to help his people in any way he could. I cannot sympathize with him and I cannot pity him. But I can feel compassion for him, and I can see how, in another situation and another time, he might have been a good man.

Taking a terrorist in our ambulance also taught me about the State of Israel and my people. The fact that the only wound on his body was a gunshot to the leg means that the soldier who arrested him did not want to kill him. They did not beat him up, nor was he underfed or tortured. He was in perfect health aside from the leg injury, and the soldiers treated him very well. At no point did I feel angry at the behaviour in the ambulance; the soldiers acted so humanely that I wanted to hug each of them. My faith in the possibility of justice was strengthened incredibly by that ambulance ride. I love this country.

This year in Israel has been the greatest learning experience for me; not only have I learned so much medicine, I have become a stronger, better person. The person I really am is being revealed to me in bits and pieces every day, more so than ever before. It's a beautiful thing, learning to know oneself, to find one's strengths and limitations. I hope to continue on this track throughout the rest of my life, starting August 13 with the beginning of medical school. But I don't think I could ever in my life learn more than I feel I have this year.

I have been present and treated people at three births, one CPR, two bombings, and countless other interesting and not so interesting calls. I have treated police, terrorists, soldiers, politicians, homeless people, Jews (from secular to Haredi), Arabs, tourists, you name it. So many individuals have entered my life and left "footprints on my heart" as the poem goes.

I will never be the same girl I was when I first came here last June, nor do I want to go back to that state of being. I feel so much more fulfilled now, so much more educated. I feel more open and at the same time more closed, more hopeful and at the same moment in despair. My heart is full but empty, my soul is flourishing and destitute. I feel like one big contrast, and I am grateful for that feeling. It means I am alive.

I am coming back to Canada on July 28; I'll send more emails then.

Love

Sara

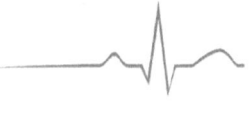

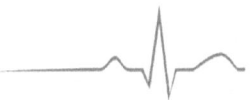

40
Epilogue

Leaving Israel was the most difficult decision I had yet made in my young life. I had the option to start medical school in either Montreal, with my family, or in Be'er Sheva in the south of Israel. Ultimately, as you know, I chose to come back to Montreal, and by doing so, I cemented a life outside of Israel. I never made aliyah, and have only been back to Israel once since the end of the period in which this book takes place. That one return trip was to celebrate Yudah's wedding, and in the process, I became engaged to the love of my life. He proposed on one knee at the Kotel, sealing my heart to his in the heart of Jerusalem, which is the heart of the land that still holds a large piece of my heart. I now practice as an Emergency Physician, and continue to write about the patients I see, the stories I become a part of, and the incredible realities of life as it dances around me.

The friends and family I wrote about in this book live thousands of miles away, across the ocean, but their faces and the laughter, tears and moments we shared remain vivid in my mind. I hope at least some of you are reading this, and that I have done justice to the experiences we lived together. You shaped me into the woman, physician, mother and strong, independent person I am today, and for that I thank you. This book is a tribute to all of you; to your strength, fortitude, resilience, and ability to find joy in the midst of underlying constant stress. The lessons I learned from the peoples of Israel will buoy me throughout my life, and I endeavour at every opportunity to instill these values in my children. *Am Israel Chai*!

Please join me along the rest of my journey, as this series of books continues through medical school, residency, and into the life of an attending Emergency Physician. I promise you a roller-coaster of emotions, including delight, wonder and enchantment, while also diving to the depths of sorrow and injustice. You will witness anger, resentment, confusion, and a loss of faith — but then I hope we will rebound together into a new understanding, grace, and ultimately peace.

Thank you from the bottom of my divided heart, for travelling back in time with me to the place and time where I stood side by side with heroes. There and then, I took my first proper steps into medicine, and into the rest of my life.

Dr. Sara Ahronheim, BScH, MDCM, FRCPC-EM

March 2, 2022, Hotel Quintessence, Mont Tremblant

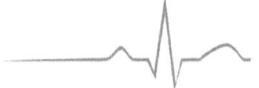

Glossary of Terms

Adrenaline and **atropine** - lifesaving resuscitative medications used to try and get the heart to start or pump more effectively.

Agunah (singular) / ***Agunot*** (plural) - women who live in limbo because their husbands refused to give them a Get when they separated. These women cannot remarry under Jewish law, and cannot move on with their lives.

Aish HaKodesh - holy fire

Aliyah - literally, ascending. Moving to Israel is referred to as "making Aliyah", because one is ascending to the Holy Land.

Ambu - bag-valve-mask device

Am Yisrael - the Nation of Israel, the Jewish People

Aran - multi-casualty incident, like a terrorist attack or multi-vehicle car accident

Ariel Sharon - former Prime Minister of Israel, elected in 2001

Ascherman Chest Seal - special one way valve dressing that allows air out but not back in. Used to prevent the worsening of a pneumothorax, where air escapes the lung and gets trapped around it, causing compression of the vital structures.

Atan - Mobile ICU ambulance, staffed by an EMT and paramedic. Provides advanced life support and first aid.

Azrieli Towers - complex of skyscrapers in Tel Aviv

Bagging - ventilating; giving breaths using a bag-valve-mask device called an Ambu

Balagan - ruckus, chaos, mess

Bat (singular) / **Bnot** (plural) **Sherut Leumi** - National Service volunteers. Individuals who, at the age of eighteen, choose not to participate in the mandatory army service (for religious or other recognized reasons) and instead participate in an internship (National Service) for two years.

Bat Mitzvah - coming of age ceremony for Jewish girls, when they are considered to be full members of the community. Once reaching Bat Mitzvah, girls are responsible for their own actions whether by performing the commandments (Mitzvot) or sins.

Beit Din - Jewish court of law. In Israel, these are a part of the formal legal system and must be consulted for some ritual matters such as divorce and conversion.

Beit HaMitnadev - "clubhouse" for the youth volunteers at MDA Jerusalem

Beit HaNassi - official residence of the President of Israel

Ben Yehuda Street - central shopping district in Jerusalem with tourist shops, restaurants and more. Sadly this has also been a nexus for terror attacks.

Beshert - literally, destiny. Often used in sentences to mean soulmate, the person one is divinely destined to marry.

"Biglal Haruach" - inspirational song by Shlomi Shabbat. The title means, literally, "Because of the spirit". Please see:

>https://www.youtube.com/watch?v=JsEgNb6O_Fo

>https://www.youtube.com/watch?v=Hium-xajVNc

Bnei Akiva - religious Zionist youth movement

Burekas - Sephardi or Israeli baked stuffed pastry, filled with a variety of things such as potato, cheese, spinach and more. Turkish origin.

Cardiopump - compression-decompression device used to assist in CPR

Cervical collar - rigid device that goes around a patient's neck to prevent worsening of spinal injuries

Chag Sameach - happy holidays - traditional greeting on a holiday

Challah - traditional Jewish braided egg bread eaten on Shabbat

Chamsin - oppressive, hot, southerly, sandy wind full of dust, arising from North Africa in spring and summer. From the Arabic *khamsin*, meaning fifty (in Hebrew, fifty is chamishim). These weather phenomena appear approximately fifty days of the year, which is where the name comes from. Even though it sounds like the Hebrew word for hot (*Cham*), this is not the origin of the word.

Chanukah - Jewish holiday commemorating the victory of the Jewish army, called the Maccabees, over the Greeks who had destroyed the Temple in Jerusalem and forced the Jews to convert under pain of death. We celebrate a miracle, when the Jews found one small pot of oil in the ruins of the Temple and it somehow kept the candelabra (menorah) lit for eight days. On the modern holiday of Chanukah we light a menorah with eight candles, using a ninth one called the shamash. Each night the shamash is used to light one more candle, until on the final night all eight are lit.

Chanukiah (singular) / ***Chanukiot*** (plural) - similar to menorah, candelabra lit on the holiday of Chanukah

Chayei Sara - chapter of the Torah, recounting the death of Sara, Abraham's wife, and the meeting of Isaac and Rebecca (Abraham and Sara's son and eventual daughter-in-law).

Chesed - loving kindness

Chevrah - group of friends

Chevruta - literally, fellowship - a style of traditional Jewish learning whereby a pair studies a topic together. These pairs often study in one big hall called the *Beit Midrash* (study hall), and the sounds of dyads in discussion fills the air. This creates a very unique atmosphere that is inspirational and warm.

Chiloni - secular, non religious

Cholent - slow cooked stew traditionally prepared before Shabbat, to be eaten at lunch on Saturday. Usually contains meat, potatoes and beans among other ingredients.

Chovesh - Medic

Chul - the diaspora - outside of Israel

Code Orange - Incident when multiple injured patients are being brought to the Emergency Department at once, and which has the capacity to overwhelm the resources available. For example, mass shooting, bombing, multi-vehicle car accident, chemical spill.

CPR - cardiopulmonary resuscitation - attempts to restart the heart once it stops

Dati Leumi - Religious Zionist Jewish sect

Daven - pray

DOA - dead on arrival

Druze - Middle Eastern religious sect, living mostly in Lebanon, Syria and Israel. In Israel they number around 150,000 and live in the north. They are loyal to the State of Israel, and Druze soldiers have fought in the Israeli army during every Arab-Israeli war.

"El Maleh Rachamim" - literally, God full of compassion. Memorial prayer, traditionally recited at funerals, when visiting the grave of a loved one, during memorial services, and more. Sung in a haunting chant. Please see:

https://israelforever.org/gallery/music/el_malei_rachamim/

Emunah - faith, belief

EMT - Emergency Medical Technician

Eretz Israel - Hebrew for the Land of Israel

Exodus ship - ship that carried Holocaust survivors to Israel, only to be denied entry by the British. The ship was actually sold for scrap, and purchased by the Haganah (underground Jewish military group) in 1947. 4500 displaced persons and survivors, from children to elderly, were transported from France to Israel only to be forced back by the British to camps in Germany.

Falafel - Middle Eastern street food consisting of balls of crushed, fried, seasoned chickpeas eaten in a pita or laffa bread, accompanied by different kinds of salads and sauces.

Galil - Hebrew for the Galilee - fertile, mountainous region in Northern Israel covered in green trees and flowers. The cities of Tzfat (Safed), Tiberias and Akko (Acre) are found here.

Galut - The diaspora, exile, where Jews were dispersed after the Temples were destroyed

Gemarah - part of the Talmud, with more commentaries and elaboration of oral law

Get - literally, divorce. This is a document orthodox Jewish men must give their wives in order to make a divorce official.

Golan Heights - most northern reaches of Israel, at the border with Syria. A mountainous region, containing the only ski hill in Israel (Mount Hermon). Was part of Syria until 1967, when Israel took the area during war in order to guarantee the safety of it's citizens who were being fired upon constantly and indiscriminately by Syrian forces since 1948 (the first Arab-Israeli War).

Haftarah - selection of portions from the book of Prophets, chanted after the Torah portions are chanted on Shabbat. The Torah and Haftarah have distinct "trope", or musical notes, written on each word, and learned by the individuals who sing these in synagogue.

Har - mountain

Har Herzl - Mount Herzl, site of Israel's military cemetery and of Yad Vashem, the Holocaust memorial. The annual official ceremonies for *Yom Hazikaron* and *Yom Ha'atzmaut* take place here. It is the final resting place for Israel's leaders and heroes. Har Herzl is named after Theodore Herzl, founder of modern Zionism, the movement to re-establish the Jewish homeland in Israel.

Haredi - Ultra-Orthodox Jewish sect

Hashem - Hebrew word for God, literally means "the name"

Hasidim - Jewish ultra-Orthodox sect

Havdalah - the ceremony separating the Sabbath and the days of the week, consisting of four prayers often sung together in a beautiful rendition once three stars can be seen in the sky on Saturday night. A candle made of braided wicks is held aloft, a strong fire burning, while the prayers are chanted over wine, fire, and the aroma of spices. It is a beautiful way to end one week and begin a new one.

Hayalim Bodedim - Lone Soldiers - soldiers whose parents do not live in Israel

Hefetz Hashud - suspicious object, for example, a package left on a road, that could be a bom

Hillel - the largest Jewish student organization in the world, made up of branches at over 550 colleges and universities

Hishtalmut - literally, "continuing education"; training session at MDA

Hypoglycemia - state of having a low blood sugar; this can lead to seizures

ICU - Intensive Care Unit

IDF - Israel Defense Forces - the army of the country of Israel. In Hebrew, Tzahal.

Intifada - rebellion, uprising - in this book it refers to the period from 2000-2005, known as the second intifada. This was a period of intense Palestinian violence against Israelis.

IV - intravenous tubing that allows delivery of medications and fluids into the veins of a patient

Jay Peak - ski hill I grew up skiing at, in Vermont

Kabbalat Shabbat - the prayers to welcome in the Sabbath, recited as a congregation on Friday evening

Kaddish - prayer for the dead

Kalaniyot - anemone flowers

Kartissiya - Israeli bus pass

Keren Kakement Le'Israel - Jewish National Fund - KKL-JNF is Israel's largest environmental organization, and the oldest one in the world. It was founded in 1901 and has planted more than 240 million trees in Israel, amongst many other endeavours.

Kibbutz - collective, traditionally agrarian community unique to Israel. These operate by the rule that all income generated goes into a communal pool; there is a specific social contract based on egalitarian and communal principles.

Kiddush - traditionally, a small meal after prayer services, opened with the prayers over wine and bread

Kikar Rabin - Rabin Square, renamed for Israel's Prime Minister Yitzhak Rabin, who was assassinated here in 1995. It was formerly named Kings of Israel Square. Situated in Tel Aviv, it was the site of many political demonstrations and rallies. On November 4, 1995, Yitzhak Rabin gave a speech at a rally for peace and was then murdered at this site. That speech is now engraved on a marker in the square.

Kikar Safra - Safra Square, in Jerusalem. Houses the municipal buildings, and is a popular spot for folk dancing, festivals and demonstrations.

Koach - strength

Kol Hakavod - literally, "all due respect", or well done

Konnanim - volunteer medics who carry pagers and respond to ambulance calls in their area

Kotel - also known as Wailing Wall, Western Wall. The last remaining wall of the ancient Jewish temple complex. It is where traditionally notes are placed asking for help from God. Prayer services are held here multiple times per day, as well as Jewish ceremonies.

Kugel - a traditional baked casserole usually made of a starch such as potatoes or noodles, mixed with eggs and oil. Jerusalem Kugel is a unique dish made with egg noodles, caramelized sugar and black pepper, and is often served at Jerusalem synagogues after prayers on the Sabbath.

Lachatz - pressure, stress

Lag Ba'Omer - Jewish holiday celebrated on the thirty-third day of counting the Omer. The Omer is the forty-nine day period between the holidays of Passover (the exodus from Egypt) and Shavuot (when the People of Israel received the Ten Commandments at Mount Sinai). This holiday is traditionally celebrated with bonfires, picnics and weddings. The rest of the Omer is supposed to be a more subdued time and a period of cleansing to prepare for receiving the Torah on Shavuot. According to the Talmud, during the Omer, a plague decimated thousands of students of the great Rabbi Akiva because they had not been respectful to one another. On the thirty-third day, the plague ended, and no one else died. Additionally, Rabbi Shimon Bar Yochai, the author of the Zohar (text of the Kabbala, Jewish Mysticism) died on Lag Ba'Omer and before he passed away he instructed his students to celebrate this day as one of joy.

Lailah Tov - goodnight

Lavan - white ambulance, staffed by medics and EMTs who provide basic life support and first aid

"Leorech Hayam" - song by Ofra Haza. Literally, along the seashore. Lyrics include "tell me how to stop the tears", "tell me how to live with death, hiding the tears every night". Please see:

    http://hebrewsongs.com/?song=leorechhayam

    https://www.youtube.com/watch?v=G1GdI1qI1ZY

Livui - army escort. Usually at least one jeep full of soldiers, that accompanied the ambulance into dangerous areas.

Machane Yehudah Market - open air market in Jerusalem, where shopkeepers sell aromatic spices, nuts and dried fruits piled in pyramid shapes. Here you can find all sorts of fresh produce, baked goods, and more as well as restaurant stalls.

Ma'apilim - An overnight activity held every summer at Camp Massad, a religious Zionist summer camp in the Laurentian Mountains outside Montreal. In the middle of the night, without alerting the campers beforehand, counsellors wake kids up and make them dress in dark clothing, forcing them out of the bunks and into the forest. This "game" reenacts the way Jewish refugees arriving in Israel after the Holocaust, had to hide and run through darkness to avoid being captured by the British and returned to Europe. The kids at camp were taken in groups by a counsellor, running through the dark forest silently to arrive in "Israel" - a bonfire at one extreme of the camp land.

Ma'ariv - evening prayer service - one of four daily prayer services in Judaism

Machsom - military checkpoint

Magav - Israeli Border Police

Magen David - Star of David

"Mah Avarech" - song written by Rachel Shapira, memorializing Eldad Kruk, a soldier in the IDF who was killed during the 1967 Six Day War. Literally, "what shall I bless him with?". Please see:

https://israelforever.org/programs/remembering_israels_fallen/with_what_shall_i_bless_him/

Matzav - literally, situation. Term used to refer to the security reality in Israel.

Mayanot - synagogue in Nachlaot, Jerusalem, founded in 1998

MCAT - Medical College Admissions Test - exam that every aspiring student has to take in order to be considered for medical school. Some schools don't require this, but the majority do.

MDA - Magen David Adom, Israeli national ambulance service. Hebrew for "red star of David".

Mechitzah - curtain or barrier separating men and women, who do not pray together in Orthodox Judaism

Memugan - bulletproof

Menorah - candelabra with seven branches for seven lights. This has been a symbol of the Jewish people for thousands of years.

Mercaz Harav - Dati Leumi yeshiva, founded in 1924 by Rabbi Abraham Isaac Kook and located in Jerusalem. One of the most prominent yeshivas in the world.

Meuleh - Hebrew - great, awesome

Mimaamakim - literally, "from the depths". The opening of Psalm 130. It begins, "Out of the depths I cry to you, Lord."

Minchah - afternoon prayer service

Mishtalem Nehigah - driver in training

Miskenah - poor thing

Mitzvah (singular) / *Mitzvot* (plural) - Jewish laws or commandments, also interpreted as good deeds

Moked - dispatch

Moshav - type of village in Israel which is a cooperative agricultural community

Motzei Shabbat - the end of Shabbat, when the sun sets and a new day begins

Muezzin - person who calls Muslims to prayer at the mosque five times daily

Nachal - river, stream

Nargila - water pipe, also known as shisha or hooka. This is used to smoke flavoured tobacco, most often around a circle with others.

Natan - Mobile ICU ambulance, staffed by an EMT, paramedic and physician. Provides advanced life support and intensive care such as intubation, chest tube insertion, and lifesaving medications.

Nefilah - nuclear/chemical/biological warfare incident

Neshama (singular) / *neshamot* (plural) - soul / souls

Neshek - weapons

Nesiah Dchufah - urgent ambulance call, lights and sirens

Nevi'im - biblical book about the Prophets

Nifgaei Terror - literally, injured by terrorism. Term used to describe not only direct victims of attacks, but also their friends and families who are indirectly touched by terrorism.

OD - overdose

Old City of Jerusalem - ancient walled area of Jerusalem, comprising sites holy to the three major religions (Christianity, Islam and Judaism), as well as residential areas.

Passover seder - traditional meal held on the evening of the holiday of Passover. This holiday celebrates the exodus of the Israelite slaves from Egypt thousands of years ago. The seder can go on for hours, and usually large groups gather to celebrate together.

Pesach - Passover - celebrating the exodus from Egypt. An eight-day holiday during which Jews do not eat leavened bread, because when the slaves escaped from Egypt they did not even have time to let their bread rise.

Pigua - terrorist attack

Pikud Eser - individual in charge of first response at the scene of a multi-casualty incident

Rabbi Shlomo Carlebach - a famous Hasidic Jewish musician and Rabbi. His joyful and catchy tunes are regularly chanted at synagogue.

Rechov - street

Refuah Shlemah - literally, full recovery, or more loosely translated as speedy recovery — what we say to people who are sick or injured

Rikudei Am - literally, national dancing, or folk dancing

Rosh Chodesh - the first day of the new month in the Hebrew, lunar calendar

Rosh Hashana - Jewish New Year. Apples dipped in honey are traditionally eaten to symbolize a sweet start to the next year.

Ruach - spirit, for example, when kids at a summer camp sing with spirit

Rugelach - a type of delicious pastry sold warm and gooey in big boxes in the markets

Sabra - term that is used to describe any Jewish person born in Israel. The Sabra fruit is also known as prickly pear — a cactus fruit with a thorny outside but a soft, sweet, delicious centre. The typical Israeli Jew is often described similarly — a rough exterior, but a kind heart.

Saying Tehillim - the act of reciting specific Psalms from the book of Tehillim. Many religious Jews do this in order to pray for specific things, or to memorialize someone.

Schacharit - morning prayer services

Schnitzel - fried chicken cutlet

Shtick - literally means comic or repetitive performance, but slang used as crap — as in, sick of their shtick = sick of their crap.

Seudah Shlishit - literally, third meal. A light meal eaten on Shabbat afternoon.

Shabbat - the Jewish Sabbath, the day of rest, celebrated from Friday at sunset until one hour after sunset on Saturday (or by tradition, until you can see three stars in the sky).

Shabbat Shalom - traditional greeting on the Sabbath, meaning "peaceful Sabbath".

Shabbat Shalom U'Mevorach - have a peaceful and blessed Shabbat

Shakshuka - Middle Eastern and North African dish, traditionally eaten for breakfast, consisting of poached eggs in a spicy tomato sauce

Shaliach - an Emissary of the Aliyah Movement at the Jewish Agency, working overseas to help connect Jewish communities to Israel

Shalom - Hebrew word that is typically used as a greeting for both hello and goodbye. Literal translation is "peace".

Shavua Tov - traditional greeting after the Sabbath is over, literally "good week", as in "have a good week"

Shekel - Israeli currency

Shema Yisrael - most important prayer in Judaism, affirming the monotheistic nature of the religion. Traditionally recited twice a day, as well as often taught to children to say before bed and for people to recite as their last words before death. Often felt to be a comfort.

Sherut - shared taxi, often a large minivan, usually crammed with passengers

Shipudim - skewers of meat cooked over a grill — common street and restaurant food in Israel. Often basted in different marinades, or rubbed with aromatic spice mixtures.

Shir Chadash - synagogue in Jerusalem, founded in 2000. Literally, a new song.

Shira Chadasha - name of another synagogue in Jerusalem, founded in 2002. Progressive, emphasizing a larger role for women in synagogue life. Literally, a new song, but feminine.

Shkiah - dusk

Shlepping - moving slowly, carrying heavy baggage

Shtachim - areas of Judea and Samaria, on the West Bank of the Jordan River. Of great historical significance to the Jewish people, this region holds the final resting places of our ancestors such as Abraham, Sarah, Isaac, Rebecca, Jacob, Rachel and Leah. Tradition holds that they are buried in Hebron. Bethlehem is the birthplace of King David, and Nablus (known as Schechem in the Torah), is where Jacob and his family settled. This region is hotly contested but the Jewish people have long, strong roots here.

Shuk - outdoor market

Shul - synagogue

Talmud - central text of Rabbinic Judaism. It is a compilation of ancient teachings and interpretations of Judaic laws and customs.

Targil - Hebrew, meaning exercise, practice

Tefillah - prayer

Tehillim - the book of Psalms

Tekes - ceremony

Tikvah - hope

Tisha B'Av - day commemorating all the awful things that have happened to the Jewish people in the last two thousand years (the destruction of the two Temples in Jerusalem, the Spanish Inquisition, and more). This is a twenty-five-hour fast day, without food or water, spent in prayer and contemplation.

Tiyul - trip, field trip, excursion

Torah - the Jewish bible made up of five books, telling the stories of creation and of the Jewish people

Tremp - hitchhike — surprisingly, a relatively common way of getting around Israel, notwithstanding the dangers.

Tut / tutim - mulberry/ies

Tzfat - the ancient city of Safed, centre of Jewish mysticism (Kabbalah)

UIA - United Israel Association

Wadi - dry river valley

Yad Lebanim - organization delegated by Israel to commemorate the fallen soldiers, and support their families

Yakar - small congregation in Jerusalem, literally means dear, precious, costly

Yerushalayim - Jerusalem

"Yerushalayim Shel Zahav" - literally, Jerusalem of Gold. Written by Naomi Shemer and sung beautifully by Ofra Haza. A song about longing for Jerusalem, at that time under Jordanian occupation. Jews had been banned from the city and had lost their homes and possessions, and yearned to return. Please see:

https://israelforever.org/interact/multimedia/yerushalayim_shel_zahav/

Yeshiva - school for religious Jewish studies

"Yihyeh Tov" - song by David Broza. The title means "Things will get better". Please see:

>https://www.youtube.com/watch?v=EvWZutHb2ZI

Yishuv - settlement, village

Yoledet - woman about to give birth

Yom Ha'atzmaut - Israel's Independence Day

Yom Hazikaron - Israel's Memorial Day, commemorating both fallen soldiers and victims of terrorist attacks

Yom Yerushalayim - Jerusalem Day - the anniversary of the liberation and unification of Jerusalem, in 1967 during the Six Day War. This day marks the first time in thousands of years that the entire city of Jerusalem came under Jewish sovereignty.

Za'atar - Middle Eastern spice usually made up of a mixture of oregano, thyme and/or marjoram, with sumac and sesame seeds

Zaka - a religious organization formed in 1989 with the original purpose being to respond to terror attacks and ensure all the body parts were retrieved, identified and buried. Has grown now into a humanitarian organization providing search and rescue, mortuary, canine and other services in over fifteen countries.

Zionism - Jewish nationalist movement with the goal to create and support the State of Israel. Zion is an ancient name for this land. Zionism as a movement originated in eastern and central Europe in the mid-nineteenth century; in fact, my family members were a part of this group and helped to found the city of Rishon LeZion ("first to Zion").

Index of Piguim Mentioned

Beit Shean pigua - Two Palestinian men carried out a grenade and shooting attack at a polling station for elections, in the city of Beit Shean, on November 28, 2002. Six people were killed and thirty-four injured. The Al-Aqsa Martyrs Brigade claimed responsibility.

Dolphinarium pigua - June 1, 2001, at the Dolphinarium discotheque in Tel Aviv, a suicide bomber affiliated with Hamas blew himself up at the entrance. Twenty-one young people aged fifteen to thirty-two were brutally murdered, mostly new immigrants from the former Soviet Union. One hundred and thirty others were wounded.

Hebrew University pigua - bombing of the cafeteria at the Hebrew University, on July 31, 2002. This attack was perpetrated by Hamas; eight students were killed and over eighty more wounded. The terrorists responsible and their families were paid over $1 million in "pay for slay" payments.

Itamar pigua - Attack on the settlement of Itamar in 2002. Two Palestinian terrorists broke into the settlement at night and entered a home, where they murdered a mother and three of her children, wounding two other children. A security guard was also killed while trying to rescue the family, and the house was set ablaze. The Popular Front for the Liberation of Palestine (PFLP) claimed responsibility.

Karkur Junction pigua - Suicide bombing at the Karkur Junction near Hadera, on October 21, 2002. A jeep driven by two young Palestinian men and loaded with one hundred kg of TNT rammed into the back of a stopped passenger bus, exploding and killing fourteen people, wounding another fifty. The Al-Quds Brigade, the military arm of Palestinian Islamic Jihad, claimed responsibility.

Kenya attacks - on November 28, 2002, terrorists in Mombasa, Kenya coordinated two attacks on Israelis. First, they fired surface-to-air missiles at an Israeli passenger jet, but missed. Minutes later, three suicide bombers blew themselves up outside an Israeli-owned hotel, killing 14 people and wounding many more. A group in Lebanon calling itself The Government of Universal Palestine in Exile, The Army of Palestine, claimed responsibility.

Mike's Place pigua - Mike's Place is a bar in Tel Aviv. On April 30, 2003, a British Muslim man blew himself up in a suicide bombing at the entrance, where young people were lined up for a fun night out. He killed three people including the bouncer, Avi Tabib, who had managed to stop the attacker from entering the packed interior. A second bomber escaped and later drowned in the sea. Hamas and the Al Aqsa Martyrs Brigade claimed responsibility for the attack.

Otniel Yeshiva pigua - terrorist attack in 2013, when two Islamic Jihad terrorists broke into the kitchen of the religious boys school and murdered four students. The heroic actions of Noam Apter and the other three boys, who had locked the doors between the kitchen and dining hall, saved the remainder of the students (over one hundred) from certain death while sealing their own horrific fates.

Rechov Yafo pigua - suicide bombing on city bus #14, in the heart of downtown Jerusalem, on June 11, 2003. Seventeen people were killed and over one hundred wounded. Hamas claimed responsibility for this devastating attack.

Sonol gas station pigua - double suicide bombing on October 27, 2002, at a gas station at the entrance to the settlement of Ariel. Two young men blew themselves up, killing three people and injuring eighteen others. Hamas claimed responsibility for these murders.

About the Author

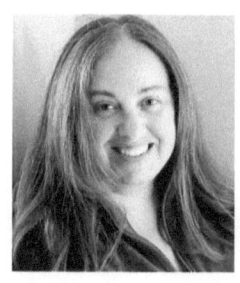
Dr. Sara R. Ahronheim is an Emergency Physician trained at McGill University. She currently works in a large academic hospital located in Montreal, Quebec, Canada. Aside from patient care, Dr. Ahronheim teaches medical students and residents how to become compassionate, knowledgeable physicians. She also runs the Physician Wellbeing program at her site, and is passionate about maintaining work-life balance and promoting joy at work. An alumnus of Queen's University, Dr. Ahronheim studied Wildlife Biology there while dipping her toes in medicine as a volunteer with the First Response Team.

Dr. Ahronheim blogs at myblackscrubs.com, where she often posts short essays about experiences in the Emergency Department. She has had stories published in the Canadian Journal of Emergency Medicine (CJEM) as well as in many other journals, newsletters and websites.

Dr. Ahronheim is a mother to two wonderful, rambunctious children and a lovable tiny goldendoodle. Married to the love of her life, Elie, for the last fourteen years, she enjoys spending winter date nights in the backyard hot tub and summers out on a nearby lake.

For photos, updates and more please see http://saraahronheim.com.

www.ingramcontent.com/pod-product-compliance
Lightning Source LLC
Chambersburg PA
CBHW030036100526
44590CB00011B/223